Maximizing Life

Maximizing Life

in the Midst of Pain and Suffering

by Linda Snook

This book is lovingly dedicated to my precious husband, Doug, who has faithfully and patiently traveled with me through my pain journey. He has shared each up and down, each step toward improvement, and each set back. Without him I would not be where I am today.

Table of Contents

Acknowledgements

*M*y thanks to the many skilled and caring medical professionals who are not mentioned specifically in this book, but who have shaped its contents as well as my life. I thank you for teaching me many of the lessons and strategies I describe in these pages, and for supporting me as I worked others out for myself. Specifically, I want to thank Karol Andrew for her wise and willing advice, and also for her skillful and compassionate treatment that has spanned so many years.

Many thanks to my family and friends, who have walked with me through my pain journey and have helped me in so many ways. In particular, my thanks to Lynda Lindsey for giving me so much of her time and encouragement at a very critical point in my life. I thank my parents, Ann and Gary Langer, for their unending love and care, and for instilling in me the character traits that have helped me adapt to the challenges of my life. Thanks, too, Mom and Dad, for being on the proofreading team.

Thanks to those of you who cheered me on through the years I spent writing this book. Special thanks to Sheila Groel for her expertise and dedication as my editor.

Finally, I thank my Lord Jesus for making every day good, regardless of the circumstances.

Foreword

This book is the fruit of my personal pain journey. For years I wanted to write down what I was learning about God in the midst of my pain, but I hurt far too much to focus my thoughts enough to get them on paper. (Not to mention that at that time it was physically impossible for me to type more than a few paragraphs at a sitting.) However, I was able to verbally share my thoughts with people God sent my way who were struggling with pain. Encouraging them to embrace God and His plan for their life in the midst of their trials also helped me.

I became more and more convinced that God is not squeamish about pain. He uses it freely in our lives for His good and loving purposes. My life was transformed by learning to meet God in the midst of my pain rather than just asking Him to end it. I pray that God will help you embrace Him in the midst of your pain.

You will find many scripture verses written out in this book. Although it is best to look them up in your own Bible, I have found it valuable to also be able to look at verses side by side. It is amazing to see what all God has to say on the subject of pain and suffering. Verses that describe God's purposes for pain and suffering are spread throughout the Bible. I have gathered many of them together here to make it easier for you to examine the scope of God's plans for you in the midst of your suffering.

My prayer for you is that you will seek to know God better in the midst of your pain and suffering and allow Him to reveal His purposes to you as you learn to rest in Him.

Linda Snook
Lawton, Oklahoma 2010

Part One

Establishing a Solid Foundation

*L*earning to live life with pain and suffering as constant companions is much like climbing a mountain. It is an uphill journey! Yet hiking and mountain climbing are very popular sports, so that indicates that there must be a way to enjoy the journey.

One very important element of hiking or mountain climbing is the terrain. Hiking is pleasant when there is solid ground underneath you. If it is steep it may be necessary to go slowly or to use switchbacks, but with good pacing it is still fun. However, when slippery mud, wet and slippery rocks, or loose and unstable gravel are under your feet, the journey quickly becomes nerve-racking instead of fun. The steepness of a climb is more manageable than is unstable footing.

This is an important point to grasp as you travel the often-uphill journey of life with pain. A solid foundation under you will enable you to make progress on your journey. The first part of this book is devoted to establishing a solid foundation. Your ability to travel through the journey of life will depend largely on the quality of this foundation.

Chapter 1

Perspectives on Pain and Suffering

*A*s Americans of the 21st century, we live in a sleek and streamlined society. We expect life to go well for us. With all the Internet availability, fast foods, and drive-thru conveniences, we expect it to happen quickly! When a problem arises we expect it to end quickly because we have a life to get on with. Therefore it comes as no surprise that most Americans see pain as a problem to be solved, an annoyance that should be quickly resolved.

For people in many other societies, pain and suffering are the norm. They are simply evidence of life. People pray for strength and endurance to get them through , rather than focusing on praying for them to end. Pain, suffering, and death are daily issues. Overcoming pain and suffering provides a big part of the meaning of their daily existence.

God's Perspective on Pain and Suffering

So then, what is God's perspective on pain and suffering? We see in the Old Testament that God's plan was for the Israelites to live comfortable and prosperous lives in the

Promised Land that He provided for them. He promised to bless them *if* they would honor and obey Him. But as they enjoyed the "good" life God had given them, they got caught up in the worldly blessings and forgot to honor and obey Him. Then, when their lives fell apart because they weren't living as God had instructed them to live, they returned to Him, crying for help. He intervened and saved them. They became comfortable in their prosperity once again and returned to their disobedient ways. So God sent another enemy or disaster of some sort to give them opportunity to remember Him and to turn back to Him.

This provides some food for thought. God desires to provide for you, but He desires even more that you honor Him and obey Him with all your heart. Are you staying close to God in your relative prosperity? Are you honoring and obeying Him? Whenever problems come your way it is wise to turn to God first, not only for help but also to search your soul and see if you are living in obedience to Him.

In the Bible we also find many people who stayed close to God for most all of their lives–David, Noah, Abraham, and Solomon, to name a few. Were their lives free from trials and suffering just because they were faithful to God? No! Their lives were full of suffering and trials too. God used those difficult circumstances to draw them even closer to Him, to help them experience how powerfully He could work on their behalf, to reveal the depth of His love and faithfulness to them and to the people around them, and to continue to conform them into His image so that others could see God in them.

God's goals for your life

It seems, then, that trials and suffering may be just as much a part of God's plan as are comfort and prosperity. Is this true? If prosperity and comfort aren't God's main goals for your life, what goals would He have you aim for? God provides many goals for you in his Word. Here are just a few of them.

> **Deuteronomy 6:5 (NIV)** Love the LORD your God with all your heart and with all your soul and with all your strength.
>
> **John 13:34-35 (NIV)** "A new command I give you: Love one another. As I have loved you, so you must love one another. By this all men will know that you are my disciples, if you love one another."
>
> **John 14:23 (NIV)** Jesus replied, "If anyone loves me, he will obey my teaching. My Father will love him, and we will come to him and make our home with him.
>
> **John 17:32 (NIV)** I in them and you in me. May they be brought to complete unity to let the world know that you sent me and have loved them even as you have loved me.
>
> **John 6:29 (NIV)** Jesus answered, "The work of God is this: to believe in the one he has sent."
>
> **Matthew 5:14-16 (NIV)** "You are the light of the world. A city on a hill cannot be hidden. Neither do people light a lamp and put it under a bowl. Instead they put it on its stand, and it gives light to everyone in the house. In the same way, let your light shine before men, that they may see your good deeds and praise your Father in heaven.

Instead of aiming for prosperity and comfort, God offers the goal of loving, believing, honoring, and obeying Him no matter what your circumstances happen to be. Then, as you live through difficult circumstances with the assurance that God is with you and working on your behalf in the midst of your difficulties, the people around you will see how God's promises "light" your path and give you hope. Your hope is in something greater than pleasant circumstances. It is in a God who can work good from any circumstance.

The Westminster confession offers some good insight when it says that the chief end of man is to enjoy God and glorify Him forever.   As you walk with God through life's circumstances and deepen your relationship with Him, you enjoy your friendship with Him.   You glorify God as you patiently and confidently trust that He is in the midst of your pain and suffering.   Your purpose might have been to live a prosperous and comfortable life, but God had a higher goal for you: to glorify Him in whatever circumstances you find yourself in.

Pain—the Master Sculptor's Tool

As hard as it may be to comprehend, pain is actually a tool in God's hand.   He does not use it only to get your attention or to punish you. He uses it to shape and perfect you. He uses it quite often, but always very carefully, tenderly, and precisely. He painstakingly sculpts you with it, shaping you into His image.   Each bit of pain reveals one more bit of detail in the sculpture.   It is very helpful to remember this as you deal with pain in your life and in the lives of others.

Your pain is not pointless.   God is actively working in your life through it. It would make no sense to try to knock the chisel out of the sculptor's hand as he is creating a masterpiece, just because you want to prevent him from damaging the marble.   There is a plan and a reason for each piece the sculptor chisels away.   Likewise, God is accomplishing something with each bit of your pain and suffering.   So it is counterproductive for you to focus your prayers and thoughts simply on ending any pain that comes your way. You can and should pray for relief and for strength to endure, but at the same time you can be watching for the sculpture of your life to take shape.

If you are willing to look at your pain and suffering from God's perspective, you will see some amazing things. God uses pain and suffering in many ways. They draw you closer to Him because they give you reason to need His help. Oddly enough, this allows you to get to know Him better and to enjoy His presence. You can enjoy *Him* even though you aren't enjoying your undesirable circumstances. Others will notice the strength, hope and joy that result from your enjoyment of God. You will be showing them God, which is what it means to glorify God. But there is more, much more that God is doing in your life through pain and suffering. He is also shaping, molding, and perfecting you to conform you to His image.

Adopting God's Perspective on Pain and Suffering

Once you begin to see pain and suffering as a tool in God's hands rather than something to be avoided at all costs, you will see evidence of how God uses pain and suffering all through the pages of scripture and in the world around you. Here are just a few verses that bring to life God's plan for pain and suffering.

Deuteronomy 18:15,16 (NIV) He led you through the vast and dreadful desert...to humble and to test you so that in the end it might go well with you.

2 Corinthians 1: 8-9 (Msg) It was so bad we didn't think we were going to make it... As it turned out, it was the best thing that could have happened. Instead of trusting in our own strength or wits to get out of it, we were forced to trust God totally.

James 1:3-4 (Msg)   You know that under pressure, your faith-life is forced into the open and shows its true colors. So don't try to get out of anything prematurely. Let it do its work so you become mature and well-developed, not deficient in any way.

1 Peter 4:12-13 (Msg)   Friends, when life gets really difficult, don't jump to the conclusion that God isn't on the job. Instead, be glad that you are in the very thick of what Christ experienced. This is a spiritual refining process, with glory just around the corner.

Pain and suffering are not things to look forward to. You certainly don't need to seek them out.   But when they come your way, rather than making it your top priority to end them or avoid them, view them as opportunities to draw closer to God. Expect God to perfect and to complete you through them.

Adjusting your Perspective on Pain and Suffering

As you seek to adopt God's goals for your life, it helps to refocus on Him, instead of on your pain and suffering. This will give you a positive focus while you are in the midst of your problems. As you read the following scripture verses, ask God to help you adopt the attitudes described in each passage.

Expect trials
Know that trials and suffering are a normal and necessary part of life.

1 Peter 4:12, 13 (NIV)   Dear friends, do not be surprised at the painful trial you are suffering, as though something strange were happening to you. But rejoice that you participate in the sufferings of Christ, so that you may be overjoyed when His glory is revealed.

Draw near to God and cooperate with him.

Turn yourself and your circumstances over to God just as soon as you see trouble on the horizon. Also stay close to Him when things are going well.

Psalm 27:1,5,13-14 (NIV) The LORD is my light and my salvation— whom shall I fear? The LORD is the stronghold of my life— of whom shall I be afraid? For in the day of trouble he will keep me safe in his dwelling; he will hide me in the shelter of his tabernacle and set me high upon a rock. I am still confident of this: I will see the goodness of the LORD in the land of the living. Wait for the LORD; be strong and take heart and wait for the LORD.

Trust in God's love for you

Know that God loves you dearly. He does not enjoy seeing you suffer. He will not allow any unnecessary suffering, only what is necessary to complete what He is working in your life.

Lamentations 3:25-26,32-33 (NIV) The LORD is good to those whose hope is in him, to the one who seeks him; it is good to wait quietly for the salvation of the LORD. Though he brings grief, he will show compassion, so great is his unfailing love. For he does not willingly bring affliction or grief to the children of men.

Know that God is in control of everything

Know that God is sovereign. These difficulties haven't happened by mistake or while God's attention was elsewhere. God has a plan for you and this is part of it.

> **Colossians 1:15-17 (NIV)** He is the image of the invisible God, the firstborn over all creation. For by him all things were created: things in heaven and on earth, visible and invisible, whether thrones or powers or rulers or authorities; all things were created by him and for him. He is before all things, and in him all things hold together.
> **Romans 8:28 (NIV)** And we know that in all things God works for the good of those who love him, who have been called according to his purpose.

Seek to glorify God and enjoy Him forever

Wait expectantly for God to work on your behalf. Seek to honor God through your situation. Seek comfort, strength, endurance, and hope from Him every day. You can enjoy God even when there is nothing else to enjoy.

> **Philippians 4:4 (NIV)** Rejoice in the Lord always. I will say it again: Rejoice!
> **2 Corinthians 12:9-10 (NIV)** But he said to me, "My grace is sufficient for you, for my power is made perfect in weakness." Therefore I will boast all the more gladly about my weaknesses, so that Christ's power may rest on me. That is why, for Christ's sake, I delight in weaknesses, in insults, in hardships, in persecutions, in difficulties. For when I am weak, then I am strong.

Let your hope rest in God, not in things of this earth

Know that God is pleased by your faithfulness. He is looking forward to rewarding you, when you get to heaven and in heavenly ways here on earth.

James 1:12 (NIV) Blessed is the man who perseveres under trial, because when he has stood the test, he will receive the crown of life that God has promised to those who love him.

Psalm 19:14 (NIV) May the words of my mouth and the meditation of my heart be pleasing in your sight, O LORD, my Rock and my Redeemer.

Know that God will multiply good from your suffering

Remember how Jesus had to suffer to complete God's plan for His life, and how that suffering has blessed you. Know that God will work much good from your suffering for you, for others and for His kingdom.

2 Corinthians 1:3-4 (NIV)   Praise be to the God and Father of our Lord Jesus Christ, the Father of compassion and the God of all comfort, who comforts us in all our troubles, so that we can comfort those in any trouble with the comfort we ourselves have received from God.

Remember that God's ways of doing things are a lot different from yours! (See Isaiah 55:8-9.) You won't fully understand God's ways until you get to heaven. But you can *learn* about His ways from what He tells you in His Word. As you get better acquainted with His ways they won't surprise you quite so much. As you adopt His goals, you will find it much easier to follow His ways because you will both be headed in the same direction.   Then, as you begin to walk more comfortably in step with Him, you will enjoy His presence and experience His joy and peace more and more. The beauty of all this is that the joy and peace you find in Him can be with you always! It doesn't come and go with your circumstances. It is with you in the midst of any and all circumstances if you simply maintain your relationship with Him. Enjoying God in the midst of your circumstances is a worthy goal for living!

Chapter 2

God's Word on Pain and Suffering

*I*s it God's plan for you to suffer? Most of us prefer to avoid this question altogether. We just hope and pray that God will protect us from pain and suffering. However this very attitude leaves us unprepared to deal with pain and suffering when it comes our way. So let's see what we can learn from God's Word about His role in our pain and suffering.

We all have our own opinions and questions about God's role in our suffering and pain, but what is *God's opinion* about it? Let's look at God's Word and learn from it what *God* has to say about His role in our pain and suffering.

Resist the temptation to skip over or just skim the verses throughout this chapter. Once you understand them, these verses will actually be a soothing balm for you in the midst of pain and suffering. God's Word is living. It is much more than just a history book or a set of rules. If you read His Word expecting to converse with Him in the same way you converse with a friend, you will find that God does "speak" to you through His Word. Verses (or parts of verses) may stick in your mind. A new meaning for a verse may come to mind as you read it. These are ways that God speaks to you through His Word.

This is your opportunity to find out firsthand what God says about pain and suffering. Take your time as you read these verses. Read God's Word expecting to listen to Him and to learn about His perspective. Reading the verses out loud may help you to "listen" better. Also, have a highlighter or pen handy to mark passages that stand out.

Psalm 71:20(NIV) Though you [God] have made me see troubles, many and bitter, you will restore my life again; from the depths of the earth you will again bring me up.

Isaiah 45:7(NIV) I form the light and create darkness, I bring prosperity and create disaster; I, the LORD, do all these things.

John 16:33(NIV) "I have told you these things, so that in me you may have peace. In this world you will have trouble. But take heart! I have overcome the world."

Romans 8:17(NIV) Now if we are children, then we are heirs --heirs of God and co-heirs with Christ, if indeed we share in his sufferings in order that we may also share in his glory.

Philippians 1:29(NIV) For it has been granted to you on behalf of Christ not only to believe on him, but also to suffer for him,

1 Peter 4:19(NIV) So then, those who suffer according to God's will should commit themselves to their faithful Creator and continue to do good.

These verses may not be consistent with the picture you have in your mind of God. We read here that God makes you see troubles, He gives you adversity and affliction, He creates disaster, and He brings grief. What happened to your loving God? You may have completely overlooked such verses over the years without considering what God is telling you in them.

Purposes for Pain and Suffering

If God is in your pain, if He plans to work through it, it would be helpful to have a clear idea of what He is up to. It is easier to endure trials when you know where they are heading. You can make it your goal to not simply get to the end of the trial, but to watch for signs that you are still headed the right direction.

As you focus your thoughts on wisdom from God's Word, it will be like a road map. It will help you to see where God is leading you on your pain journey. Watch for refinement in your character. Watch for God to cover you with His compassion. And watch for spiritual and emotional healing as well as for physical healing.

If you are only looking for a quick end to your problems you may overlook some amazing sights God has planned for you to see. God will work good in your life through pain and suffering in many ways.

We are going to look closely at two of those ways right now. Take your time as you read the verses. Underline the parts that help to explain some of God's purposes for suffering in your life.

Pain and suffering mature and complete you.

God disciplines you, matures you, and makes you more productive through your trials. Your faith needs testing to develop. It is really only a theory or idea until you have had an opportunity to live it out. When you find yourself in the middle of a difficult situation, you have the opportunity to cling to the truths you have learned from God's Word. In faith you say, "This is not hopeless because God has promised to be with me and to provide for me. I can't see or feel His presence at the moment but I choose to believe that what He has said is true. God, be with me and guide me through this storm." When the difficulty subsides you find that your faith has been strengthened. When the next trial comes, you can say with even more confidence, "God will get me through this too."

Psalm 116:6-7 says, "When I was in great need he saved me. Be at rest once more, O my soul, for the Lord has been good to you." This psalm shows us how the psalmist experienced this very truth. The psalmist could rest in his confidence in the Lord to see him through his present trouble because God had taken care of him in previous problems. The testing of your faith makes it stronger, just as pottery must be fired to become strong, durable, and truly useful.

> **Psalm 119:67,71 (NIV)** Before I was afflicted I went astray, but now I obey your word. It was good for me to be afflicted so that I might learn your decrees.
>
> **Proverbs 17:3 (NIV)** The crucible for silver and the furnace for gold, but the LORD tests the heart.
>
> **John 15:2 (NIV)** He cuts off every branch in me that bears no fruit, while every branch that does bear fruit he prunes so that it will be even more fruitful.
>
> **Romans 5:3-5 (NIV)** Not only so, but we also rejoice in our sufferings, because we know that suffering produces perseverance; perseverance, character; and character, hope. And hope does not disappoint us, because God has poured out his love into our hearts by the Holy Spirit, whom he has given us.
>
> **Hebrews 12:7 (NIV)** Endure hardship as discipline; God is treating you as sons. For what son is not disciplined by his father?
>
> **James 1:2-4 (NIV)** Consider it pure joy, my brothers, whenever you face trials of many kinds, because you know that the testing of your faith develops

perseverance. Perseverance must finish its work so that you may be mature and complete, not lacking anything.

God's aim is to strengthen and mature you. Only mature plants and trees bear fruit. Only fired pots can withstand the rigors of daily use. So when the fire and growing pains become intense, instead of letting your thoughts linger on the heat and pain, rejoice that soon you will be stronger, more mature and able to bear fruit for God.

Pain and suffering draws you closer to Jesus.

It is important to seek God out in your times of need. He intends to help you, to guide you, to provide rest for you, and to have you rely fully on Him. But He doesn't push himself on you; He waits for you to seek His help.

2 Corinthians 1:9-10 Indeed, in our hearts we felt the sentence of death. But this happened that we might not rely on ourselves but on God, who raises the dead. He has delivered us from such a deadly peril, and he will deliver us. On him we have set our hope that he will continue to deliver us,

Psalm 28:7 The LORD is my strength and my shield; my heart trusts in him, and I am helped.

Psalm 73:23-26 Yet I am always with you; you hold me by my right hand. You guide me with your counsel, and afterward you will take me into glory. Whom have I in heaven but you? And earth has nothing I desire besides you. My flesh and my heart may fail, but God is the strength of my heart and my portion forever.

Psalm 130:5 I wait for the LORD, my soul waits, and in his word I put my hope.

Psalm 146:3,5 Do not put your trust in princes, in mortal men, who cannot save. Blessed is he whose help is the God of Jacob, whose hope is in the LORD his God.

Isaiah 64:4 Since ancient times no one has heard, no ear has perceived, no eye has seen any God besides you, who acts on behalf of those who wait for him.

You may have been taught to be self-reliant and independent as you were growing up. You may feel that you shouldn't trouble God with your problems, that you should be able to deal with them yourself. This makes it hard to ask God for help. The "I'll do it myself" attitude is not supported by these verses. It is important that you work hard and keep trying, but God wants you to do it by depending on Him, not on your own strength.

If you are a parent, you may have had the experience of watching your child do something by himself when you would have liked very much to help, to offer advice, or just to be with him during the experience. Your heart ached to be a part of his life. Yet if he is determined to do it himself, you are excluded. How often does God feel that way about you? Seek His help. Include Him in all of your life. Know that you aren't bothering Him. He wants very much to be with you and to help you in everything that you do.

Your suffering is actually a chance to discover your "poverty"–your need for Christ. You are not all-powerful. The day will come when you will reach the end of your own strength and resources. In the midst of your trials, when you are acutely aware of your need for your Savior, you have a unique opportunity to deepen your relationship with Him. You are ripe to experience His love, compassion, faithfulness, and power.

Chapter 3

Your Pain Works Good for Others

$\mathcal{N}$ow we will consider two more very significant purposes for pain and suffering. Jesus had to learn by suffering. He learned obedience and was made perfect through His suffering. All of us certainly have benefited from Christ's suffering. Should we expect to be exempt from suffering if it was so necessary in our Lord's life?

God uses your pain and suffering to encourage the people around you

It was God's will to use suffering in Jesus' life to benefit you. Therefore it seems reasonable that God will use suffering in your life for the benefit of the people around you.

Hebrews 2:10 (NIV) In bringing many sons to glory, it was fitting that God, for whom and through whom everything exists, should make the author of their salvation perfect through suffering.
Hebrews 5:8-9 (NIV) Although he was a son, he learned obedience from what he suffered and, once made perfect, he became the source of eternal salvation for all who obey him.

Hebrews 12:2(NIV) Let us fix our eyes on Jesus, the author and perfecter of our faith, who for the joy set before him endured the cross, scorning its shame, and sat down at the right hand of the throne of God.

2 Corinthians 1:3-6 (NIV) Praise be to the God and Father of our Lord Jesus Christ, the Father of compassion and the God of all comfort, who comforts us in all our troubles, so that we can comfort those in any trouble with the comfort we ourselves have received from God. For just as the sufferings of Christ flow over into our lives, so also through Christ our comfort overflows. If we are distressed, it is for your comfort and salvation; if we are comforted, it is for your comfort, which produces in you patient endurance of the same sufferings we suffer.

2 Corinthians 4:6-11(NLT) For God, who said, "Let there be light in the darkness," has made us understand that this light is the brightness of the glory of God that is seen in the face of Jesus Christ. But this precious treasure—this light and power that now shine within us —is held in perishable containers, that is, in our weak bodies. So everyone can see that our glorious power is from God and is not our own. We are pressed on every side by troubles, but we are not crushed and broken. We are perplexed, but we don't give up and quit. We are hunted down, but God never abandons us. We get knocked down, but we get up again and keep going. Through suffering, these bodies of ours constantly share in the death of Jesus so that the life of Jesus may also be seen in our bodies. Yes, we live under constant danger of death because we serve Jesus, so that the life of Jesus will be obvious in our dying bodies.

We tend to serve others out of our plenty. We volunteer in those areas where our natural strengths lie (rightly so, as we can do the best job there.) We give out of our relative abundance (compared to the rest of the world.) It is right and good that we share the bounty that God has given us. But there is something more God may give you the opportunity to do. He may allow you to share from your weakness, not just from your strength.

Through pain and suffering, God may strip you down, past your layers of abundance, your strengths, abilities, cheerful personality, financial security, etc., to the point where you are exposed and vulnerable and not at all eager to show yourself, much less share yourself with the world around you. Yet here, from your weakness, God's strength can best be seen in you. Because when others have seen you suffer, they are inclined to think you might relate to their situation and might be of some help to them. If you seek God's comfort in your times of need, you will be able to pass on to others what they truly need–that same comfort that you received from God.

As you endure pain and suffering, you have the opportunity to glorify God.

As you rely on God and draw from His strength in your pain and suffering you glorify Him. The people around you get to see God at work in your life. You are a showcase that displays who God is and how He works in your life. When you trust God and look forward to your heavenly hope (especially when there doesn't seem to be any other hope), people notice. They can see the hope in your attitude and in your actions. They tend to wonder why you have hope, given your situation. You can still smile, enjoy the people around you, and care about others because you know that God cares about you and He has your situation well under control.

1 Peter 1:6-7 (NIV) In this you greatly rejoice, though now for a little while you may have had to suffer grief in all kinds of trials. These have come so that your faith -- of greater worth than gold, which perishes even though refined by fire --may be proved genuine and may result in praise, glory and honor when Jesus Christ is revealed. **Philippians 3:8,10-11(NIV)** What is more, I consider everything a loss compared to the surpassing greatness of knowing Christ Jesus my Lord, for whose sake I have lost all things. I consider them rubbish, that I may gain Christ... I want to know Christ and the power of his resurrection and the fellowship of sharing in his sufferings, becoming like him in his death, and so, somehow, to attain to the resurrection from the dead. **2 Corinthians 4:16-18 (NIV)** Therefore we do not lose heart. Though outwardly we are wasting away, yet inwardly we are being renewed day by day. For our light and momentary troubles are achieving for us an eternal glory that far outweighs them all. So we fix our eyes not on what is seen, but on what is unseen. For what is seen is temporary, but what is unseen is eternal. **Romans 8:17-18 (NIV)** Now if we are children, then we are heirs --heirs of God and co-heirs with Christ, if indeed we share in his sufferings in order that we may also share in his glory. I consider that our present sufferings are not worth comparing with the glory that will be revealed in us.

God is giving you a very powerful ministry. As the medical professionals and other patients around you observe your hope, they will take notice. They are quick to notice people with hope and peace, because most pain patients lack these qualities. Everyone in the office can be encouraged by the peace in your heart and the smile on your face that goes with it.

You may even get an opportunity to share a bit about God's goodness and why you have hope in Him.

Also, sharing in the common ground of suffering with Christ allows you to know Him in a way that can only be accessed by suffering. When you walk through a difficult time with the Lord by talking to Him and relying on Him, you emerge from that time with a deep and precious bond with Him. Your time of suffering allows you to appreciate in a new way how He suffered for you. It is humbling to realize how much He endured to pay for your sins. Having just a small taste of suffering compared to what He endured allows you to cherish and honor Him all the more. This gives you the opportunity to realize more fully the greatness of His love for you. You can share your appreciation of Him with the people around you through your words and your attitude.

Trust God even when you don't understand Him

It seems fairly clear from these passages from God's Word that He plans to use pain and suffering in our lives. But why would our good and loving God include pain and suffering in the box of tools He uses to shape His beloved children? God tells us in Isaiah 55:8-9 that His ways are beyond our understanding. Certainly this subject helps to prove that point. We will never fully understand why God does what He does until we are with Him in heaven. However it helps to search His Word for glimpses into His nature and His way of doing things, so that we won't be so surprised at some of the things that happen to us.

You can trust God even if you don't understand Him. You can rest in His promises and know that He is not only working on your behalf in every situation you find yourself in, He is working *good* on your behalf. Focus on God and His goodness, rather than on the less-than-good circumstances you may experience. This will greatly reduce the stress that those circumstances cause you. You may never fully understand why some things happen, but you can grow in your depth of understanding of the goodness, mercy, compassion, gentleness, strength, and faithfulness of the God who carries you through those circumstances.

Reflecting on God's nature offers you insights that can't necessarily be gained by trying to understand God's ways. In closing, here is a poem that I hope will help you to see God's nature reflected in pain and suffering.

The Christmas Jewel
by Linda Snook

A lowly stable, surrounded by poverty and suffering,
    in the midst of a fallen world.
What a perfect setting for the Christmas Jewel!

Unending needs display the marvel of His sufficiency.
Pain and suffering highlight the beauty of His comfort.
Injustice and inequity reflect the hope of His unconditional love.
All of these perfect the setting where the Christmas Jewel rests.
It is here that the fullness of His glory is most clearly seen.

He is the One who was intended to satisfy the longings of your soul.
He is the One who can bring peace into your life and into the world.
He is Truth, Love, Life and Light -- for this world and especially for you.

This Christmas, open the Gift that God sent you.
Enjoy the splendor of the Christmas Jewel.
Let Him be the jewel of your life. Receive Him, wear Him,
    let Him be a part of all you are and do.
Let His wisdom, strength, joy, hope, patience,
    peace and provision guide and sustain you.
May their beauty be reflected in every corner of your life.

May the Christmas Jewel be the jewel of your life,
    this year and for eternity.

Chapter 4

A Closer Look at God

*I*t will be helpful for you to take a break from the pain and suffering that looms so large in your thoughts, and to focus on something that is even bigger—God. As you improve in your understanding of God, you will strengthen the foundation that supports all you are and all you do. Building a relationship with God involves connecting to and depending on the One who has infinitely greater strength and abilities than you do. As you begin to trust God and depend on Him and His resources, rather than depending only on yourself or those around you, you will find that your own strength and abilities will become less and less of an issue. God's strength and abilities are truly sufficient to meet all of your needs.

This is very much like learning to ride a bike. At first it seems unnatural and risky to balance yourself over two wheels and let them roll you down a street. You may prefer walking to the uneasy feeling of being out of control. But once you learn to work with the bike, it is a joy and at times even a thrill to sail down a hill or to fly past pedestrians. It takes some effort and determination to learn to rely on wheels instead of legs to move, but it is worth the effort. The same is true about learning to rely on God instead of on yourself to move through life. It isn't natural or easy, but it is very well worth the effort.

Your picture of God

The starting point for this adventure is in comparing two different pictures of God–yours and His. Some people view God as a kind of Santa Claus. They give Him their wish list and then judge how good they have been by how much of the list God gives them. Other people see God as a taskmaster who has written an impossible list of rules that He expects them to follow. God is also viewed as the creator of the universe who, after finishing His creation, sits back and watches it unfold. There are also those who see God as their loving father, whose arms are always open to welcome them.

How do you picture God? Can you think of a person who, at least to some degree, is a picture of God to you?

Now list some adjectives that describe what God is like in your opinion. This might include words like friendly, loving, vengeful, forgiving, unforgiving, or distant. Just think about God and see what words come to mind.

Now round out your picture of God by considering how you think God views you. How do you think He would introduce you to someone?

If you looked up and saw God sitting in the room with you as you were reading this book, what would you do? Run to Him? Run away? What would you say to Him? What would He say to you?

The picture you just formed of God is probably based partly on truths and partly on untruths. All the ideas seem true because you haven't necessarily stopped to consider if they are accurate or not. That is the point of this exercise–to discover any misconceptions you might have of God that could hinder your relationship with Him. For instance, if you see God as a

Santa Claus, but He really isn't, it is better to understand who He is than to be disillusioned when He doesn't act the way you expect Santa Claus to act.

God's picture of himself

Now it's time to take a look at how God pictures Himself. Fortunately, God has given you His Word, the Bible, which is a great source of information. As you read the following verses, see if you can discover (according to God,) what kind of God He is.

God's dimension and sphere of influence

In this first set of verses, look for answers to questions about the magnitude and sphere of influence of God. What role does He play in the universe? How big is He? How long has He been in existence? Is there any other being like Him?

Nehemiah 9:6 (NLT) You alone are the LORD. You made the skies and the heavens and all the stars. You made the earth and the seas and everything in them. You preserve and give life to everything, and all the angels of heaven worship you.

Job 36:26 (NIV) How great is God—beyond our understanding! The number of his years is past finding out.

Psalm 90:2(NLT) Before the mountains were created, before you made the earth and the world, you are God, without beginning or end.

Psalm 33:13-15(NLT) The LORD looks down from heaven and sees the whole human race. From his throne he observes all who live on the earth. He made their hearts, so he understands everything they do.

Colossians 1:16-17 For by him all things were created: things in heaven and on earth, visible and invisible, whether thrones or powers or rulers or authorities; all things were created by him and for him. He is before all things, and in him all things hold together.

God's affections

In this set of verses, look for what you can find out about God's affections. Who does He like or love? Under what conditions? To what degree does He care for and love His creation? Think of the most loving person you know. How does his or her love for you compare with God's love for you as described in these passages?

John 3:16 "For God so loved the world that he gave his one and only Son, that whoever believes in him shall not perish but have eternal life.

Romans 5:8 (NLT) But God showed his great love for us by sending Christ to die for us while we were still sinners.

Psalm 86:15 But you, O Lord, are a compassionate and gracious God, slow to anger, abounding in love and faithfulness.

Psalm 89:2,14 (NLT) Your unfailing love will last forever. Your faithfulness is as enduring as the heavens. Your throne is founded on two strong pillars— righteousness and justice. Unfailing love and truth walk before you as attendants.

Psalm 103:3,11,13 (NLT) He forgives all my sins and heals all my diseases. For his unfailing love toward those who fear him is as great as the height of the heavens above the earth. The LORD is like a father to his children, tender and compassionate to those who fear him.

Zephaniah 3:17 The LORD your God is with you, he is mighty to save. He will take great delight in you, he will quiet you with his love, he will rejoice over you with singing."

God's power and authority

Now see if you can create a picture of God's power and authority. Do you see any conflict between God's loving kindness and His powerful authority?

After you finish reading this set of verses, see if you can put the ideas you gleaned from all the previous verses together into a sentence or short statement that summarizes who God is and what He is like.

Deuteronomy 32:4 (NIV) He is the Rock, his works are perfect, and all his ways are just. A faithful God who does no wrong, upright and just is he.

1 Chronicles 29:11-12 (NIV) Yours, O LORD, is the greatness, the power, the glory, the victory, and the majesty. Everything in the heavens and on earth is yours, O LORD, and this is your kingdom. We adore you as the one who is over all things. Riches and honor come from you alone, for you rule over everything. Power and might are in your hand, and it is at your discretion that people are made great and given strength. "O our God, we thank you and praise your glorious name!

Psalm 91:4 (Msg)   His huge outstretched arms protect you— under them you're perfectly safe; his arms fend off all harm.

Ephesians 3:20(NLT)   Now glory be to God! By his mighty power at work within us, he is able to accomplish infinitely more than we would ever dare to ask or hope.

Philippians 4:19 (NLT)   And this same God who takes care of me will supply all your needs from his glorious riches, which have been given to us in Christ Jesus.

Word pictures of Jesus

You may have found it difficult to come up with a concise, accurate description of God. It's no wonder. God is beyond our comprehension. It's not surprising that it is difficult to describe Him. In fact, Jesus was well aware of this problem. He chose to compare Himself to familiar, earthly things to help people grasp various aspects of His being. Since Jesus is the image of the invisible God (Colossians 1:15,) this will help us as we seek to develop a picture of God.

As you read these verses, consider the implications of each word picture for you personally. (For instance, if Jesus is my light, then when I'm "in the dark," Jesus could guide me.)

John 6:35 (NLT) Jesus replied, "I am the bread of life. No one who comes to me will ever be hungry again. Those who believe in me will never thirst.

John 8:12 (NLT) Jesus said to the people, "I am the light of the world. If you follow me, you won't be stumbling through the darkness, because you will have the light that leads to life."

John 10:11,14 (NLT) "I am the good shepherd. The good shepherd lays down his life for the sheep. I am the good shepherd; I know my own sheep, and they know me.

John 11:25 (NLT)   Jesus told her, "I am the resurrection and the life. Those who believe in me, even though they die like everyone else, will live again.

John 14:6 (NLT) Jesus told him, "I am the way, the truth, and the life. No one can come to the Father except through me.

Jesus is your bread, your light, your shepherd, your life, your way, and your truth. In other words, He has promised to nourish and provide for you; to provide warmth and direction; to guide your way, to look out for potential hazards and protect you from them; to give you life with fullness beyond what you can imagine, and to be your firm foundation of truth in all you do. This exercise has only scratched the surface of the truths expressed in these word pictures. Take some time to contemplate them one by one. Let Jesus Himself show you more of what He means by each of these images.

Chapter 5

God and You

$\mathcal{G}$od is more than just a good *guy*, he is a good, a very good *God*! How can anyone really picture God? He is a loving father, a protector, a provider. He is compassionate, kind, and loving. He is our Savior. He is too many things to fit into one picture. He sees all, He knows all, He made everything, and He has always existed. He IS! He is everything and always.

You may not have been able to form a truly accurate or all-encompassing picture of God, but what a great comfort it is to have tried to picture God. It is so easy to take Him for granted and to never really consider all that He is.

If you don't know much about His greatness, you won't ask or expect Him to help you in the great ways that He is capable of working in your life. You can't rest in His care for you if you don't know that He is great enough to take care of your every need and concern.

What a good feeling it is to know that someone, who is in every way great beyond description, cares so very much for you! Remember all that He is. Accept the fact that you won't be able to fully understand Him because He is too much for a human to truly comprehend. But rejoice in this fact! Don't let it frustrate you. Think of how very capable that makes Him to meet all of your needs.

In the days and weeks to come, make an effort to remind yourself that God is who *He says* He is, not who *you think* He is. Expect Him to act as He says He will act. Ask Him to help you let go of your old expectations of Him. Ask Him to help you to trust Him. If there are some very significant discrepancies between your picture of God and His picture, it may be worth your while to discuss them with someone you trust and respect spiritually.

God in the midst of your circumstances

Now that you have, fresh in your mind, a sense of God's greatness, His goodness, and His control over all the universe, it's time to turn back to where we started–your pain and suffering. Hopefully your own personal trials will not seem quite so ominous after considering God and His incredibly great capacity provide and care for you. No problem is problematic for Him. He could resolve any or all of your problems in a second. But as you have already seen, He uses your problems to complete His purposes for your life and the world around you. Rather than just ending your trials, God's intent is to walk with you, to comfort you, to carry you when needed, to encourage you, and to let you deepen your relationship with Him as you travel with Him through them.

Are you willing to meet God on His terms and seek to stay connected to Him as you walk through the challenges of each day? He has so very much He wants to give you and be for you. You may be mad at Him or disappointed in Him because of something that happened to you or a loved one. You may be harboring bitterness or lack of forgiveness toward God or someone else. You may prefer to do things yourself rather than asking anyone for help, including God. Or you may want God to help you enact the plan that you have in mind. All of these situations will distance you from God and all that He intends to be for you. Instead of resting in His total sufficiency and letting Him guide your path, it's easy to limit God to what you want from Him. He could force Himself on you, but as the loving father that He is, He doesn't. Instead, He let's you chop away at your picture of Him until it fits the shape that you want Him to have.

Big God or big problems? Where is your focus?

As you limit God (in your mind's eye) to less and less of the fullness of who He is in order to suit your purposes, your problems will tend to seem bigger and bigger. God will no longer be the biggest thing in your sight: your problems will be. Why? Because you chose to focus on and value most highly something other than God. You may have put your plans above Him or your bitterness or anger. You may have cherished your independence or your sense of self-accomplishment about your faith in God. You may have decided that your situation is hopeless, that it is beyond what even God could or would help you with. Or you may simply have chosen to agree with the "wisdom" of the world around you rather than trusting God.

You have a choice to make on a daily, moment-by-moment basis—you can choose to believe God and enjoy Him in all His fullness, or you can turn from Him to other things. You can come to Him, learn to be "yoked" to Him (to walk in step with Him), and allow Him to carry the weight of your burdens, or you can strive to make it alone or with help that comes from somewhere other than God. You can trust Him and find Him to be trustworthy. You can depend on Him and find Him to be faithful. Or, you can treat Him as if He were less than all that He has told you that He is. You can bargain with Him, ignore Him, or turn your back on Him. The choice is yours. But if you chose anything other than God in His fullness, you will miss experiencing "His mighty power at work within us, able to accomplish infinitely more than we would ever dare to ask or hope." (Ephesians 3:20)

God is so great, so infinitely greater than any of your problems. Why limit yourself to human-sized resources when God has offered you His God-sized resources to deal with your problems? Just like learning to ride a bike, it is worth taking the effort to learn to depend on God instead of limiting yourself to your own resources.

God's Perspective on your problems

How do you keep God foremost in your thoughts when you are surrounded with the problems of this world?   By adopting God's perspective on your problems.   God says that once you have become a child of His by inviting Him into your heart, you are no longer a citizen of this world. Instead you are a citizen of heaven and a member of His heavenly household. For the present you still live on the earth, but now you are a foreigner here.   Someday your visa will expire and you will go to your true home–heaven.   How does this affect your daily concerns and worries? It gives you a new perspective on them. When you are done with your stay on earth these things won't matter at all!   So it is important not to allow them to spoil the days you have on this earth.

Our earthly problems can be compared to the problem of losing your luggage at the beginning of a long-awaited trip. You can either pick up what you need to continue on with the trip, or you can spend days trying to locate the luggage and let its loss cloud your attitude for the rest of the trip. The point is that the trip will only last for so long. Yes, you envisioned it without difficulties, but you can have a wonderful time regardless of the difficulties, if you keep your focus on the goal of enjoying each day you have. In the end you may even find that your memories are more special because of the difficulties and how you adapted to them. At any rate, you will go home to your house full of belongings, and the inconvenience of the lost luggage will fade into history. It was far more important to focus on making the most of the trip than on the difficulties that arose.

Focusing on Eternal Things

God says, in Matthew 6:33, that if you will seek Him above all else, your needs will be met. Unfortunately, it is more natural to deal with what you see around you–your material needs–than to make God your highest priority. So it is necessary to take time to refocus on God and His kingdom, and to let all the problems that press in around you fade a bit. Eternal things like God and His kingdom will be a part of your life forever. It is wise to invest your time and energy in them (not to mention the fact that God commands you to do so.) Your earthly troubles press hard right now, but they will be gone soon enough. Don't let them spoil the days that the Lord has given you on this earth.

This may be a new way of thinking about your daily concerns. Try it out. Ask God to help you stay focused on Him. Marvel in His greatness. As you think of Him, expect to be refreshed. Look past your problems and fix your gaze on who God says He is. Your problems will still be there, but as you face them with God foremost in your thoughts, they shouldn't make your blood pressure rise quite as much.

God is capable of seeing you through your problems. Read His Word and seek to follow the counsel He gives you there. He tells you to trust Him. That may seem impossible. Ask Him to give you the strength and patience to do it. He tells you to give up your grudges, bitterness, and lack of forgiveness. Ask Him to help you keep your gaze steadily fixed on His forgiveness of your sins as you struggle to let go of the offenses others have committed against you. All this isn't easy. But it leads to immeasurable blessings.

Enjoying God's greatness in the midst of your problems

You will always have God with you and you will always have some sort of problem with you (until you get to heaven, of course!) The question is, which one will you allow to dominate your thoughts? If you place the two side by side, God will always be bigger. It is not possible for you to have a problem that is bigger than He is. But if you look at it from the wrong perspective, the problem will seem bigger. If you notice this happening to you, readjust your perspective. Focus your mind's eye on the picture of God you formed based on who He says He is in His Word.

Write down some key verses on an index card and keep them with you so that you can use them to help you readjust your focus when it starts to wander. Fix your eyes on God and let your problems shrink back down to the way that He sees them. God is the answer to all your problems–He will carry you through them until He resolves them. Fix your eyes on God and enjoy His greatness regardless of what your circumstances are like! He is great enough to see you through them.

Chapter 6

Connect With God

$\mathcal{H}$opefully by now you believe that God cares about your problems and is key in answering them. But how do you transform this belief into reality in your daily life? You live in the world and are bombarded with sights and sounds that make it difficult to stay close to God. So how do you go about walking with One whom you can't even see? How do you hear His still, small voice over the roar of the world you live in?

When you are experiencing pain and suffering (or any other kind of trial for that matter), it is easy to get upset. You may be upset at God for what has happened. You may be upset at the doctors or the insurance people, the person who caused the accident, or the circumstance that created your problem. You may be upset at everyone and hardly even know why! This is good, yes, good! This gives you an excellent starting place for learning to connect to God.

The starting place is your need. You need a healthy, constructive way to deal with the feelings that are building in you because of your pain and suffering, and the related circumstances they have brought into your life. God has promised to meet all your needs, so here is your perfect opportunity. You can learn to connect to and depend on God as you are unloading the growing burden of your trials. The growing pressure that you are experiencing can become the catalyst that helps you to develop a close and meaningful relationship with God. Take advantage of this opportunity to draw closer to God. If you don't turn *to* Him with your burdens, you most probably will end up turning *away from* Him.

Giving up your baggage

So the first order of business is to *purpose* to regularly unload your burdens on God. This is not a gripe session. This is a time to talk to God, (in other words, to pray.) You may yell, you may talk, or you may write, but the goal is to communicate to God the pressures that are building up in you, and then *leave* that baggage with Him. When you complain or gripe, you don't give anything up. You just tell your tale of woe to someone and then look for the next person you can find who will listen to your story. So rather than griping, relinquish to God the things that are bothering you. In other words, you give up your complaints and judgments about your health, your doctors, your family members, your financial situation, your boss, your coworkers, and everything else around you.

God has good plans He intends to work through the people, things and circumstances that annoy you. When you hang on to negative, critical, or judgmental thoughts about these things, those thoughts take up the space in your mind. This space could be used to consider God's perspective on these same issues and to enjoy His peace and joy in the midst of your situation. Why cling to your displeasure with your circumstances when you could be clinging to God and the good things He has to offer you?

The endless "thought loop"

One reason for clinging to these miserable thoughts is that they are so familiar it is hard to give them up. You find yourself thinking them before you even realize what you are doing.

When you think about something troublesome, whom are you addressing in your mind? You may be rehearsing the speech you would like to deliver to the person who is irritating you. You may be telling someone over and over again why your way is best or why you are right and he is wrong. You may be blaming yourself. You may be putting the words in someone's mouth that you desperately wish he or she would say, or things that you are afraid he or she will say.

Generally, thoughts like these run through your mind over and over again. There is no end to them. You rarely get the opportunity to carry out the conversations you imagine. Or if you do say those things, matters may only end up worse because you did.

Interrupting the "thought loop"

So why not try something different? As soon as you notice one of these "thought loops" running in your mind, address those thoughts specifically to God. Simply say, "God, I keep thinking about this." "Let me tell You my thoughts...". "God help me with this. Help me to learn to move on with my life despite this situation..." Whatever you say, just make sure that you are addressing God directly. Most probably you will find that in a short time you have switched back to addressing someone else and not God. Stop yourself and start telling God your feelings once again.

When you talk directly to God, the cycle that would otherwise go on and on in your mind is interrupted. He enters into that cycle and acts on your behalf according to what you request and what He knows is best for you. The first thing He usually does is to comfort and assure you that He hears you and cares about you. He will give you His peace *as you keep your mind on Him.*   He can bring thoughts to mind that are far more helpful than what you are worrying about.

You will find that talking to God is much more soothing than reliving your fears, complaints, concerns and problems. You are talking to someone who can and will make a difference in your situation. Here are a few verses that tell of God's intent to help you with your thought life and of the benefits you will experience when you keep your thoughts focused on God.

> **Isaiah 26:3 (NLT)** You will keep in perfect peace all who trust in you, whose thoughts are fixed on you!
>
> **Romans 15:13 (NIV)** May the God of hope fill you with all joy and peace as you trust in him, so that you may overflow with hope by the power of the Holy Spirit.
>
> **Philippians 4:8-9 (NLT)**   And now, dear brothers and sisters, let me say one more thing as I close this letter. Fix your thoughts on what is true and honorable and right. Think about things that are pure and lovely and admirable. Think about things that are excellent and worthy of praise.   Keep putting into practice all you learned from me and heard from me and saw me doing, and the God of peace will be with you.
>
> **1 Peter 5:7 (NLT)** Give all your worries and cares to God, for he cares about what happens to you.

Journaling is also an excellent way to express your thoughts to God. You can write to Him, telling Him about your hurts, disappointments and other feelings. Physically writing down your thoughts helps you to keep your mind from wandering. It also gives you the opportunity to look back over your thoughts at a later date. It can be very helpful to see what was troubling you a year or two ago, and how God worked in that situation.

Improved communication with God

Unloading onto God the pressures you face improves your communication with Him. This is a wonderful way to develop your relationship. You will find that even when you are mad at God you don't have to turn your back on Him. He doesn't mind if you yell at Him. He can listen to all of your unloading without taking it personally. You can yell, scream, cry, or pound your fist into a pillow. You can tell Him what has hurt you and why. The important thing is to keep talking to Him rather than turning your back on Him and shutting Him out of your thoughts.

There are times when it is not easy to keep your face toward God and communicate openly and honestly with Him. There are times when you know you have disobeyed or disappointed God. You may be embarrassed to talk to Him. You may feel that He is asking too much of you, or you may just be giving in to temptation or fleshly desires.

Determining to communicate openly and honestly with God on a daily basis provides you with the opportunity to notice early on when you are retreating from Him. Ask God to give you the desire and the determination to face Him quickly, before it becomes even harder to do so. There is a strong tendency to tell God that you will return to Him when you have your life in better order. Getting your life in order is the perfect project to work on *with* God, not apart from Him.

Guidelines for maintaining good communication with God

As you talk to God there are four areas that are important to consider. First, tell Him how you feel. Second, make your requests. Third, give the matter up to Him. Finally, thank God for listening, caring, and for being capable and willing to work on your behalf. This final step helps you to turn your thoughts away from the problem. Instead, your thoughts are on God's greatness, faithfulness, and complete capacity to deal with your issues. (Remember to talk directly to God throughout the process.) Here are some sample conversations that cover all four areas:

- ***Tell God how you feel***

God, I am going to explode. I can't take one more second of this. No matter what I do I hurt. I do what the doctor says and I hurt. I do what I want to do and I hurt. What difference does it make?

- ***Make your requests***

God, I want to feel better. Please do something to help me. Guide the doctors, guide me. Help me to really listen to you and do the things that will help... Help me to trust you and to not get so upset about this.

- ***Leave it with God***

Now, God, please take my pain problem and deal with it Yourself. My worrying about it hasn't helped anything yet and probably has made things worse. The doctor keeps telling me to reduce my stress. Worrying certainly doesn't do that. Help me to enjoy Your creation as I sit outside for a while. Please, if I can't get away from the pain, help me to take a vacation from thinking about it. May I have a nice conversation with someone? Show me someone to call...

- ***Thank God for His faithful involvement***

God, thank you for caring about me. You are so incredible, it is amazing that you care so much about me. Thank you. You are so much greater than I can imagine. Your solution to my problem is probably something I couldn't imagine either. Help me to notice your greatness in the world around me and to trust you.

The Psalms model: clear, honest communication with God

The Psalms are an excellent example of how to communicate with God. David provides us with all kinds of examples of each of these steps. He unloads all kinds of burdens on God. He has some pretty heartfelt requests for God too. He asks God to break the teeth of His enemies! He pleads with God to help him because he is afraid that he will die. David certainly maintained open, honest communication with God.

Here is a list of just a few Psalms that clearly show these four steps.

Psalm 3, 5, 13, 28, 32, 35, 40, 42, 58.

Take time to read them in the next few days. They will give you a good picture of an open, honest relationship with God. They also demonstrate how to go about staying close to the Lord in difficult times.

Note carefully what happens in these Psalms. David unloads on God, and then his negativity usually gives way to praise. David unloads his burdens on God, he makes his requests, he lets the issues rest in God's care, and then he praises God for who He is and how He works. It is important *not stop talking to God before you make it to the fourth step.* As you thank God for who He is and how He faithfully works in your life, your focus turns from your problems to God's greatness.

Rejuvenation in God's presence

After thanking God, linger in His presence to give Him a chance to talk to you. Read some Psalms or other scripture in a contemplative way. They are God's words; He will speak to you through them. Read them slowly, giving God time to bring new thoughts to your mind about what you are reading. Ask Him to help you keep your heart and mind open to Him and focused on Him as you do this. You will find that it is very soothing to your soul to get your thoughts off of your problems and onto God and His Word.

Consider God's nature. Because He is compassionate, loving, and kind, expect Him to work good in your life in the midst of your circumstances. His main goal is not to make you miserable, but to mature you, to complete you, and to fellowship with you. Believe Him. Be honest with Him. Talk to Him about any unbelief you have and ask Him to help you move past it.

Ask God to help you focus your thoughts on His promises, not on your feelings. Start memorizing verses to help you through tough moments and days. Think contemplatively on those verses and other passages of Scripture. Take time to thoughtfully consider God's love and His other wonderful attributes—His faithfulness, kindness, justice, and mercy. Consider how these characteristics of God benefit you.

You have aired your complaints, burdens, and feelings to God, but you have really done so much more. You have presented yourself openly and honestly to God and then allowed Him to respond to you. You have connected with God. You came to Him with your needs and allowed Him to minister to you. You began the relationship at your point of need. Now you can continue it anytime and anywhere. As the relationship develops, you will find yourself wanting to spend more time with God. Who knows—you may even come to the point of thanking God for those problems that gave you the opportunity to learn to connect to Him.

Chapter 7

Walk With God

$\mathcal{O}$nce you have developed some semblance of regular, honest communication with God (this will take a lifetime to fully develop), you are ready to move on to another significant element in your adventure with God–traveling with Him. In order to keep the communication going with God, it will be helpful if you are heading in the same direction as God is heading. Have you ever run a three–legged race? (This is when you race with one of your legs tied to one of your partner's legs.) A three-legged race is, in essence, a form of being yoked to someone, just as you are to be yoked to Christ. What happens if your partner decides to go a different direction from the one that you are going? To say the least, the traveling gets pretty rough! Clearly, if you want to make it to the finish line in a three-legged race, you and your partner will have to be headed in the same direction.

So what direction is God headed? God provides some very clear directions, so let's see what He says. One of the most direct comments He makes on this subject is in Matthew 6:33-34, "But seek first His kingdom and His righteousness, and all these things will be given to you as well. Therefore do not worry about tomorrow, for tomorrow will worry about itself. Each day has enough trouble of its own."

Heavenly Goals

God tell us to seek eternal things first. His instructions are that we should be headed for eternal treasures. It is fine to have earthly goals, but we should plan to let them take second place to heavenly goals. What are heavenly goals? Read the following verses and underline the heavenly goals that are mentioned.

Proverbs 3:5-6 (Msg) Trust GOD from the bottom of your heart; don't try to figure out everything on your own. Listen for GOD'S voice in everything you do, everywhere you go; he's the one who will keep you on track.

Matthew 6:19-21 (NLT) "Don't store up treasures here on earth, where they can be eaten by moths and get rusty, and where thieves break in and steal. Store your treasures in heaven, where they will never become moth-eaten or rusty and where they will be safe from thieves. Wherever your treasure is, there your heart and thoughts will also be.

Luke 9:23-24 (Msg) "Anyone who intends to come with me has to let me lead. You're not in the driver's seat—I am. Don't run from suffering; embrace it. Follow me and I'll show you how. Self-help is no help at all. Self-sacrifice is the way, *my* way, to finding yourself, your true self.

Philippians 3:8 (NLT) Yes, everything else is worthless when compared with the priceless gain of knowing Christ Jesus my Lord. I have discarded everything else, counting it all as garbage, so that I may have Christ

Colossians 2:6-7 (Msg) My counsel for you is simple and straightforward: Just go ahead with what you've been given. You received Christ Jesus, the Master; now

live him.   You're deeply rooted in him. You're well constructed upon him. You know your way around the faith. Now do what you've been taught. School's out; quit studying the subject and start *living* it! And let your living spill over into thanksgiving.
Colossians 3:1-2 (NIV) Since, then, you have been raised with Christ, set your hearts on things above, where Christ is seated at the right hand of God.   Set your minds on things above, not on earthly things.
1 Peter 1:13 (NIV) Therefore, prepare your minds for action; be self-controlled; set your hope fully on the grace to be given you when Jesus Christ is revealed.

These verses offer some challenging heavenly goals–developing your relationship with Christ, experiencing Him in every aspect of your life, learning to wait for Him, and learning to follow Him.   The development of your character is also a heavenly goal.   You will have it long after the material things around you are gone.   Letting others see Christ's presence and power in you is a heavenly goal as well.

God's will be done

Matthew 6:9-10, which is from the Lord's Prayer, offers another heavenly goal–that God's will would be done on earth as it is in heaven.   That provides quite a bit of direction–head toward God's will above your will.   His Word offers endless examples of His will.

This may seems unrealistic.   How can anyone do this?   You can't, that's the whole point!   The only way you can overlook your earthly problems and goals and choose to live for heavenly goals is through God's power.   You need Him to enable you to live as He intends for you to live.   Once again, God intends for your need to drive you to Him.

You have a choice. You can say, "This day is too bad. I am too miserable. These circumstances are too much for me. I can't overcome this. I can't possibly follow God's way here and now." Or you can say, "Lord, you have given me this day. It is too much for me, but I look to you to make it possible for me to honor you, to glorify you, and to enjoy you as I live this day. Help me as I depend on you."

Paul offers some great encouragement on this subject:

> **2 Corinthians 12:7-10 (Msg)** Because of the extravagance of those revelations, and so I wouldn't get a big head, I was given the gift of a handicap to keep me in constant touch with my limitations. Satan's angel did his best to get me down; what he in fact did was push me to my knees. No danger then of walking around high and mighty! At first I didn't think of it as a gift, and begged God to remove it. Three times I did that, and then he told me, "My grace is enough; it's all you need. My strength comes into its own in your weakness." Once I heard that, I was glad to let it happen. I quit focusing on the handicap and began appreciating the gift. It was a case of Christ's strength moving in on my weakness. Now I take limitations in stride, and with good cheer, these limitations that cut me down to size—abuse, accidents, opposition, bad breaks. I just let Christ take over! And so the weaker I get, the stronger I become.

Seek to be a good steward

In the parable of the talents (Matthew 25:14-30), Jesus shows us how important it is to God that we be good stewards of all God has given us. The master entrusted each servant with part of His wealth. He gave them a period of time to manage that wealth, expecting them to invest it and allow it to multiply. He was pleased with the servant who did so, and disappointed with the one who didn't.

In like manner, God has given each of us part of His wealth. He has given us our bodies and our lives, not to mention many material things. We are amazingly and wonderfully made. Each of us is priceless! No amount of money can buy the equivalent of any one of us. God entrusts your life to you for a period of time so that you can use it in a way that will honor and glorify Him.

You are His steward, His trusted servant, who has been given great responsibility. In fact, you may feel that the responsibility is greater than you are! That is not a reason to give up. God is willing to provide you with all the help you need. His request of you is that you use what He has given you to further His kingdom. He knows that you will face many challenging circumstances while you are His steward here on earth. He expects you to seek His help to enable you to live for His goals, rather than just giving up on them because you are afraid that you can't reach them. Here are some words of encouragement from God on that subject:

John 15:4-5 (NLT) Remain in me, and I will remain in you. For a branch cannot produce fruit if it is severed from the vine, and you cannot be fruitful apart from me. "Yes, I am the vine; you are the branches. Those who remain in me, and I in them, will produce much fruit. For apart from me you can do nothing.
Hebrews 10:22-23 (NIV) Let us draw near to God with a sincere heart in full assurance of faith. Let us hold unswervingly to the hope we profess, for he who promised is faithful.

You will discover that focusing on heavenly goals actually makes it easier to unload the burdens you accumulate on a daily basis. As you look toward and fix your eyes on God and His kingdom, you won't want to hang on to the problems of your daily life. Things that seemed enormous as compared only to other earthly things will shrink to far less significance, when placed beside heavenly goals. Heavenly goals give you the kind of motivation you need to help you let go of your earthly burdens and goals.

Enjoy God

Finally, as you *stay connected to God* through regular, open and honest communication with him, and as you *fix your eyes and mind on eternal treasures* rather than on earthly health, wealth and prosperity, you will find that a third element begins to unfold. You will find that you can *enjoy Christ anywhere, at any time, and in any circumstance.* Christ is with you and in you. You are moving together with Him toward the goal of seeing that God's will is done here on earth just as it is in heaven.

Christ is a fabulous traveling companion! He will cause you to see and enjoy marvelous things in God's creation, things to which you had paid minimal attention before–sunrises, sunsets, butterflies, birds singing, squirrels playing. All these things are happening while you are struggling with unpleasant circumstances. They give you something to enjoy in each day.

God will encourage you too.   In fact, you may find yourself talking to others who are in situations similar to yours, sharing with them some of the encouragement you have received, both from Christ's presence in you and from what you have read in His Word.

God will give purpose to your life in the midst of your struggles. You don't have to wake up to another miserable day as you may have done in the past.   Now you can wake up wondering what this new day will bring.   Yes, your pain is still there. But you can learn to work with it, work around it, and live in spite of it. There may be many things you can't do because of your pain, but as you travel through each day connected to Christ you will discover all that you can do despite the pain. If you can't even move you can still pray. You can talk to others on the phone. (You may need a hands-free phone.) You can listen to people and encourage them. Invariably the conversation will encourage you as well.

In short, you can enjoy God in the midst of your circumstances. There will always be something "wrong" with your circumstances as long as you live in this fallen world. These problems can make you miserable, but they don't have to. Even while these problems surround you, you can keep your focus on God and enjoy His infinite goodness. He may be just about all that there is to enjoy, but He is sufficient!

God is always with you, so you will always have something to enjoy. That may be the reason why Paul sang hymns in prison–he needed the lift. There wasn't much to enjoy in those miserable circumstances, but God was with him. So he enjoyed God. (See Acts 16:22-34.) Other people were blessed by Paul's rejoicing. Soon there were many people rejoicing in spite of their wretched circumstances. No wonder Paul tells us to rejoice always. He knew from personal experience that even in the most desolate of times, there is something to rejoice in because God is there.

God is the source of our joy. He is our reason to rejoice. He fills us with His joy, peace, patience, and strength as we stay connected to Him. The choice is yours. You can stay focused on earthly issues and let them drag you down, or you can learn to connect to God and enjoy Him despite the circumstances.

Part Two

On with the Hike!

$\mathcal{W}$ith the solid foundation of a strong relationship with God underneath you, it is now time to put it to the test, to see if it can give you stability as you travel through your journey with pain and suffering. In these next chapters, you will learn ways to maximize life in the midst of your pain and suffering. Just like a mountain trail, the path may seem very steep at times. But if your footing is sure, you will be able to make progress. In fact, you may even find yourself enjoying some incredible sights along the way.

If you find yourself backsliding, stop. Return to God's Word. Talk to Him about your situation. It is very difficult to implement these ideas with slippery mud or loose gravel underneath you. But with the solid foundation of God's Word and His presence with you, the journey can be pleasant, invigorating, and incredibly good!

Chapter 8

Cheap and Effective Pain Reduction

$\mathcal{Y}$ou have a readily available, cost-efficient and effective way to reduce your pain–your attitude. Your attitude toward your pain and suffering will either magnify it or diminish it. This is why the first part of this book dealt with God's plan and purpose for pain and suffering. If you see your problems as part of God's plan for you and as serving a purpose, your attitude toward your pain and suffering will be more positive. A good attitude can help you to deal more effectively with your physical problems. But can your attitude actually improve your health? Yes, most definitely, yes!

Connectedness of Body, Mind, and Spirit

It is a well-documented fact that your body, mind, and spirit are very interconnected. Problems in any one part of your being will negatively impact the other areas. By the same token, the strengths in any area will spill over and benefit the other areas too. Athletes practice guided imagery to help them perform their best physically. In a similar fashion, hypnosis and biofeedback are frequently used in pain clinics because targeting the mind can result in reductions in pain levels that medications and other therapies were not able to accomplish.

Your *attitude* is just as important as the mind-body techniques mentioned above. The way you view yourself, your body, your life, your family, and also your medical team will significantly affect your healing. You can adjust your attitude without spending a penny or driving a mile. What good news! However, adjusting your attitude is not always easy. Many people find their familiar, old attitudes to be more cozy and comfortable than their favorite old slippers. And just like those old slippers that have soles so broken down that they do the feet more harm than good, your old familiar attitudes may feel good but may actually have a negative impact on your health. With this in mind, let's look at some attitudes that could benefit your health.

Chronic pain vs. Acute pain

Some of the attitude problems concerning pain have to do with misunderstandings. One quite common misunderstanding is thinking that chronic pain is best handled in the same way as acute pain. *Acute pain* is *short-term pain, lasting hours to days. Chronic pain* is *long-term pain, lasting from weeks to the rest of your life* (more or less.) Nobody wants to have chronic pain, so it's not uncommon to assume you don't, and to simply treat your pain as if it were acute pain.

Acute pain is a warning signal from your body to pay attention and take appropriate action. That action may be as simple as getting a good night's sleep or keeping your foot up for a few hours. Or it may be a reminder to schedule a trip to the doctor or even to schedule a surgery. At any rate, with appropriate measures, acute pain decreases and goes away.

Chronic (ongoing) pain is quite different. It is not as easily gotten rid of, or else it wouldn't be chronic. It may be a result of arthritis, bone or joint degeneration, damaged nerves, diabetes, or some other health problem. It may be the result of an otherwise successful surgery. (For instance, a nerve may have been damaged during the surgery.)

Most generally, *chronic pain can be managed, but not eliminated*. This is where the misunderstanding often occurs. A common attitude toward dealing with acute pain is to ignore it until it goes away. However, this approach won't work for chronic pain because it doesn't disappear when ignored. Ignoring it and just trying to live life as before will generally cause chronic pain to worsen. It is far better to learn what things flare the pain (and avoid them), and what things reduce the pain (and practice them.) This will necessitate careful and deliberate attention to the pain, not ignoring it. This doesn't mean moaning, groaning, and complaining about the pain. Instead, it means noticing how it ebbs and flows and paying attention to which activities make it worse or better.

Attitude Adjustment

Attitudes that you have had since you were young seem like facts, they are the way you deal with life. It is hard to see how they influence you. You will need to be sensitive to God's illuminating light in your life in order to even be able to identify your attitudes. Ask Him to help you. Work on recognizing the gentle thoughts He puts in your mind to guide you.

Attitudes that accentuate the negative may be realistic in a lot of ways, but they will drag you down. There is good and bad in every situation. It is crucial to cultivate the positive when you are living with negative factors that won't be going away any time soon, like chronic pain. You need all the positive influences you can get to overcome the negatives you experience.

It doesn't work well to try to simply avoid a negative thought. The void needs to be filled with something positive or else other negative things will begin to fill it. The best way to do this is to pray as soon as you notice the negative thought or attitude. Just start talking to God. Address your thoughts directly to Him. That will interrupt the self-talk and provide some supernatural help as well.

Here is an example: "I *hate* this. I used to be able to walk as long and hard as I wanted to. Now I can hardly walk across the street. This is *hopeless*. I think I should just *give up and die*."

Rather than trying to refute each negative thought that comes to mind, just start talking to God. "God, you know that I hate this. I used to be able to do so much." (Give Him some room to speak to you, particularly through what He has said to you in His Word.)

"God, I guess you know how I feel. You allowed this to happen. You have a plan for my life. You have promised not to give me more than I can bear *with your help*. God, please encourage me. I need it. Help me to be able to walk again without pain. Show me what to do, which doctor to go to. Show the doctors how to help me. In the meantime, help me to get my mind off my pain and to be careful about what I do. Thank you for the sunshine and the birds. Help me to enjoy *you* right now. Even though I can't do what I want to do, I can enjoy you."

Talking to God does several things. First, it gets some supernatural power moving on your behalf as you ask Him for help. Next, it provides you with some major distraction from your problems. It also shifts your focus from yourself and your problems to God's view of your problems, assuming that you are willing to talk to Him about something other than your complaints. It provides you with some encouragement as you consider God's Word, and His good promises on your behalf. This conversation is much more effective than telling yourself that it is not helpful to have a bad attitude. God's Word, His presence with you and His power on your behalf can help you develop healthy attitudes.

Healthy attitudes

Here are some attitudes that will give you positive momentum so you can live a happy and productive life in the midst of your pain and suffering. Rather than dwelling on how you feel and all the activities you can't do because of how you feel, you can actively seek to develop attitudes that will help your healing process along.

Work with your pain rather than just ignoring it.

Pain is a nuisance! How well you know that. It is *hard* to live with pain. Most of us either want the pain to be gone, or else we blame it for all our problems. These aren't particularly healthy attitudes. Yes, you want the pain to be gone, but the question is, what will be your attitude towards it *until* it is gone? The serenity prayer of St. Francis of Assisi offers us a healthy attitude–*accept* that which you can't get rid of or change (at least for the present.) If you are going to have pain for a companion on your journey through life, you might as well accept its presence and learn how to get along with it.

Accepting your pain does not mean giving up on getting rid of it. It simply means that you say, "Pain is part of my life right now. How can I make the most of my life *with* this pain?" In some ways this is similar to accepting the death of a loved one. At first it seems like life can't go on without this person. But as life does go on, you work through the loss, eventually accepting the fact that you can have a meaningful life without him or her. Life will not be the same, but there is still much good in the world.

In the same way, it is necessary to work through your anger, frustration, and other feelings about your pain. It has disrupted your life. You may have lost the ability to do many things. You actually have a loss to grieve in that regard. Ignoring the pain or the loss of ability will keep you from ever accepting it. Dwelling on the loss and not moving on toward acceptance will not help you either. Identify what is happening in your life and work through it. Hopefully you will come to the point where you accept that pain has a place in your life and you'll do your best to deal with it, just as you deal with bills, family members, job decisions, and everything else in your life.

Dwell on the good.

Avoid dwelling on stressful things. Once again, every situation has both good and bad in it. If you are focused on the bad, you may miss the good altogether. Your situation may require you to consider many difficult things—pain, immobility, finances, permanent changes and losses, or choices in treatment plans. Pray and think these things through. Gather enough information to make wise decisions. However, avoid lingering on these topics beyond the point of making the necessary decisions. Dwelling on them tends to cause stress. *Stress will always increase pain.*

You can reduce your pain by reducing your stress. Make a habit of letting go of your medical concerns. Once you have come to as much of a decision as you can for the time being, turn your thoughts away from these concerns and let your mind be refreshed and renewed as you dwell on uplifting thoughts. Subscribe to *Guideposts* magazine or read other uplifting literature. Watch the kind of movies or DVDs that you find funny. Meet with a friend and agree in advance not to talk about your problems. Activities like these help you to turn your thoughts away from the stress in your life.

If it is hard for you to dwell on positive things, try making a list of positive things in your life. Then when you start to get bogged down in the negatives, you can refer to your list to help you change your focus.

The first and most important good or positive thing that we all need to let our thoughts dwell on is that *God is in the midst of our problems*. He is with you. He cares about you. When you enjoy God's goodness you always have something good to think about!   Here is just one passage that clearly speaks to this subject.

> **Philippians 4:4, 6-8 (Msg)** Celebrate God all day, every day. I mean, *revel* in him! Don't fret or worry. Instead of worrying, pray. Let petitions and praises shape your worries into prayers, letting God know your concerns.   Before you know it, a sense of God's wholeness, everything coming together for good, will come and settle you down. It's wonderful what happens when Christ displaces worry at the center of your life. Summing it all up, friends, I'd say you'll do best by filling your minds and meditating on things true, noble, reputable, authentic, compelling, gracious—the best, not the worst; the beautiful, not the ugly; things to praise, not things to curse.

God is good. If you have asked Him into your life, you are filled with good things. Read some Psalms and list some of the good attributes of God. Read the New Testament and list the many promises God and Jesus have made to provide for you in various ways.

Do you have a roof over your head? Is your room a comfortable temperature? Do you have a bed to sleep in? Many people would be thankful for any one of those things. It is natural to think about "bad" things when you feel bad, but it is not helpful. Ask God to help you keep your mind on positive things. Ask Him to give you a grateful heart and open eyes to see His goodness in every situation. Then actively seek to live out these attitudes.

Refuse thoughts of self-pity and blaming others.

These two attitudes will do more to ruin your health than many drugs will do to help it. Self-pity is a very poor substitute for the Lord's comfort and solace. He knows what it is to suffer pain, to be mistreated, to be unappreciated, to be unfairly judged, and any other form of suffering that you will ever know. He desires to comfort you in your suffering. Self-pity puts up walls between you and God, rather than allowing you to experience His comfort. It seems like He would take away the problem if He really cared, and He will–in heaven, if not before. But until He does, your suffering gives you the opportunity to share in His comfort as you share in His suffering.

God never promised anyone that life would be fair. God does promise to be with you in everything that happens to you. (Matthew 28:20b) He has promised to defend your honor. (Psalm 62:7) He has promised to give you the strength and resources you need for what ever happens to you. (Philippians 4:13,19) You have much to be thankful for–God's abundant provision, His deep and constant love, and His unfailing faithfulness–just to name a few things. Try enjoying His goodness rather than feeling sorry for yourself because of your circumstances.

Note: One of the worst things you can do for your pain problem is to be involved in a lawsuit. If you are trying to prove that someone else is responsible for your pain and suffering, you will be looking for how bad your situation is, how much difficulty someone caused you, how much your quality of life suffered, and any other possible negative that you can notice.

Many pain specialists won't take a patient if they are involved in a lawsuit. They know that they will be fighting an uphill battle. It is not worth their while to get involved, not until the legal battles are over. If you are involved in a lawsuit or other battle to prove the level of suffering you are enduring, you will need to cleanse your attitude once it is over (and as often as you can while you are involved in it.)

Expect your healing to be a process that requires significant time, attention and effort from you.

Expect to need patience and to be inconvenienced, as solutions will generally take time. Looking for quick fixes generally only causes more frustration. Advertisements on TV and in magazines tell us about pills that will quickly restore us to prime health. We do get antibiotics that can very quickly turn an infection around, but not all health problems are that quickly *cured*.

A pain pill may quickly reduce the pain for a time, but it is very important that you not confuse that with curing the problem. The source of your chronic pain has probably been developing over many years. It is reasonable that its cure (to whatever degree it is possible) will also take a significant amount of time. The problem may be the result of a series of habits and choices. The solutions will likewise require a series of adjustments to your habits and choices.

In fact, quick fixes are rarely quality fixes. They may just be cover-ups. Fixing health problems has some similarity to fixing financial problems. If you are in debt and have an acute dilemma, such as some bills that must be paid, there are different approaches to solving it. You can get another credit card and charge your bills. This will resolve the immediate issue—the bills are paid and the utilities are still connected. But this is by no means a solution. Actually, it increased the problem. Now you owe even more money.

In like manner, solving a chronic pain problem by taking more pain medication may only increase your problems down the road. There is an important place for pain medication, but careful attention needs to be given to locating and minimizing the source of the pain. This is a much slower and more tedious process, one that may require seeing a variety of practitioners.

Surgeries improve certain problems but they may cause other problems. They are not generally a perfect solution. They may be the best solution, but it is important that you realize that they may or may not restore you to the health you had before the problem began. Seeking to return to your former state may not prove to be a helpful attitude.

Make a habit of setting immediate health goals. You may not reach them immediately, but they are the next hurdles you want to overcome on your pain journey. Be specific. It is hard to know when you have met the goal of "feeling better." There is a good chance that you may never reach the goal of "getting rid of my pain." But you can give yourself something definite to work towards as well as something to celebrate by setting goals like: being able to walk 2 miles a day, going back to work at least part time or being able to drive again.

Celebrate when you reach each goal and then set a new one. As you recognize and celebrate the smaller things, such as an improvement in your ability to function in certain areas, or increased endurance, increased mobility, or improved sleep, you

build momentum to help you reach your bigger goal of having
your pain under control.

Chapter 9

More Healthy Attitudes

$\mathcal{I}$t is amazing how many readily available (and free) options you have that can improve your health. You just learned about four attitudes that can substantially reduce your pain levels. Here are four more attitudes that will also help you.

Know that you have the primary role in your healing.

Be proactive: your health is your responsibility. It is common to have the idea that your doctor is responsible for your health. If you have a health problem that won't go away, you go to your doctor. You do what he tells you, which hopefully is nothing more than taking a few pills, and soon you will be well.

But when you have a health problem that doesn't seem to be going away, what is your attitude? Do you complain that the doctor hasn't fixed you, or do you see what you can do to help the situation?

You can provide the doctor with an accurate record of your symptoms and any other information that would help him. You can pray for the doctor as well as praying for yourself. You can also look on the Internet for information that might help you live with and improve your situation.

It is true that your doctor prescribes medications for you and order procedures that help your body. But ultimately you are responsible for your body. God entrusted your body to you and He expects you to be a good steward of it. You are the bottom line as far as your body is concerned, not someone else.

Examine your attitude toward your doctors and health professionals. Do you expect them to think for you? They have ten or twenty minutes to consider your case every month or two (or however often you see them.) That is not a lot of time. They have invaluable expertise to offer you, but there is much that you need to do yourself.

You can learn to "listen" to your body and to be sensitive to what it is telling you. There are many things that you don't have to wait for a doctor to tell you. For example, if you notice that whenever you eat a large meal late at night you have heartburn after you go to bed, you can adjust your eating habits. Or, if you notice a pattern of having diarrhea after delightful trips to the ice cream parlor, you could try cutting out dairy products for a while to see if your bowels are happier.

This will require a willingness to make adjustments and modify some favorite things. You may love to work in the yard or garden on weekends, frequently ignoring your body's pleas to take a break. Or you may love to participate in recreational activities, even though they regularly cause your health problems to flare up. It is very likely that if you will listen carefully to your body and make some adjustments, you can enjoy your favorite things in modified ways and reduce your health problems by avoiding flare-ups.

Be flexible, patient, and persistent

Understand that you may have to try several drugs, several kinds of treatments, or even several medical professionals to find a good solution for your problems. Don't give up. Keep trying. Your trusted family doctor may not have the familiarity with your problem that is necessary to successfully treat you.   Medical doctors (MDs and DOs— Doctors of Osteopathic Medicine) comprise only one small segment of the full array of health practitioners that are available to you. There are many other effective ways to treat pain that are beyond the scope of a MD's normal practice.

Physical therapists are an important part of a pain management team. As they physically assess your pain problem by touching and moving your body, they often notice things that scans and blood tests don't reveal. In particular, physical therapists who use *manual techniques* can be invaluable in your quest to reduce your pain. Manual techniques manipulate soft tissues and joints to enhance mobility and function in order to reduce pain.

There are also physical therapists who help their patients return to a state of wellness by having them use machines to build strength (which resolves many problems.) Often this is not a good approach for those who suffer from chronic pain. Make sure to find a therapist who works with chronic problems, not just acute problems. (Sports rehabilitation centers may not be the best option.)

Massage, acupuncture, nutritional supplements, chiropractic, cranio-sacral manipulation, and other gentle forms of manipulation are all very effective for treating chronic pain. You should not expect your medical doctor to direct you to all these alternative treatments. He or she does not have time to study alternative treatments and keep current on all the advances in medicine too. She may be able to offer some suggestions and guidance, but MDs generally do not have a referral system in place to recommend a wide variety of alternative practitioners.

Do not expect medical doctors to have the same depth of knowledge and expertise about alternative treatments that they have about medicine, because it is not their primary field. Expect to take the initiative in exploring these options. But be sure to tell your doctor what you are doing or are interested in doing concerning alternative therapies, so that she is aware of your overall situation. She needs this information to be able to treat you to the best of her ability.

Do not be afraid of offending your doctor. It is far more important that he or she knows exactly what you are doing and what you are interested in trying than for you to never "ruffle his feathers". *It is not your job to try to please your doctor.* It is your job to be honest with him about every aspect of your situation, including telling him your preferences. Many MDs and DOs are interested in learning about the benefits their patients experience from alternative treatments. Others are not. Your doctor may acquire some valuable information from observing the results of alternative therapies you use.

You should also investigate national and local organizations that have been created to assist people with your disease or syndrome. Your doctor's office, the library, or the Internet can help you get in touch with these organizations. The Internet is an invaluable tool for learning about treatments (and ailments) and for locating practitioners. *Look for accredited practitioners who regularly work with people who have problems similar to yours.* (Ask about these things before making an appointment. The office staff should be able to provide the answers for you.) In the end, a referral from a patient who has been successfully treated is one of the best ways to locate a good practitioner.

Admittedly, this approach is not easy. It requires time, energy, and prayerful consideration. It may take trial and error, patience, and money. But the result may be a very significant improvement in your health, so do what you can and keep at it! If this is more than you can handle, look for a family member or friend who can do some advance work for you. Make sure to keep praying every step of the way. God knows far more than any of us, and He is very interested in helping you.

On the subject of doctors, it is worth mentioning the issue of *long waits* in the doctor's office. Many a potentially beneficial appointment has been ruined because the patient is out of sorts from having been kept waiting for such a long time. If you have had to wait a long time, you can assume that your doctor is just as frustrated with the schedule as you are. Do what you can to make the most of your appointment, regardless of *when* it happens. Expect to wait. Take a book. Take a pillow or a blanket or whatever you need to be comfortable. (Sometimes it is possible to call the office an hour or so before your appointment and see if they are running on time or not.) Finally, if you do want to complain, talk to the business office, not to the doctor.

Be a good reporter.

Many people are vague about their problems when they talk to their doctor. If the problem isn't manifesting itself strongly at that very moment, it is easy just to say, "Oh, I've felt a lot worse" or "I'm doing pretty well." This may be true, but it doesn't help the doctor deal with the problem that has brought you to his or her office.

Have a proactive attitude toward your doctor appointments. Do your homework and be ready to actively participate in what goes on. Have your list of medications with you. (It saves precious time that would otherwise be wasted flipping through your chart.) Be completely honest. If you have quit taking a medication (or you never started it), *say so*. If you are experiencing side effects or any kind of new symptoms or problems, *say so*. Do not wait to be asked. Do not expect yourself to remember all this. Write it down ahead of time.

Before you go to your appointment think through what you are hoping to gain or accomplish from that appointment and from working with that medical professional. Be specific. Many doctor offices actually ask you to state the primary reason for your visit and a second subject you would like to discuss if there is time. This shows the importance of carefully considering what you hope to gain from your visit.

Include in your "homework" (the written notes that you bring to your appointment) things such as:

- *The specific reason for this visit.*
- *Your immediate health goals.*
- *All the prescription and over-the-counter medications and other vitamins and supplements you are currently taking, and the dosage.*
- *Any problems or side effects you are experiencing.*
- *How you are responding to your treatment plan, especially the latest adjustments or changes.*
- *Changes in your sleep patterns.*
- *Changes in your ability to live your daily life.*
- *Changes in your digestion, diet, and eating habits.*
- *Changes in your elimination patterns.*
- *Any major health concerns.*
- *Any questions you have accumulated for the doctor since your last visit.*

The best way to gather this information is to keep a health journal. In one section of your journal, briefly describe anything significant to your health. This would include the things on the "homework" list above, and also things in the following list. (Some of these will be more relevant to your situation than others, so include those that matter the most to you):

- *Changes in the weather and how they affected you.*
- *Improvements in functionality and quality of life.*
- *Your activity levels and how you feel during and after the activity.*

- *Changes in alertness, tiredness, mood, and pain levels throughout the day. (Tracking this, along with knowing the amount and timing of your medications, may give you hints as to the effectiveness and side effects of different medications.)*
- *What you ate and how your body reacted to it.*
- *Pain levels, and what seems to reduce or increase your pain.*
- *Hours of sleep, quality of sleep, what causes you to wake up (pain, need to urinate, etc.)*
- *Any new or unusual symptoms or problems.*
- *Any major changes in your life or changes in your stress levels.*

In another section of your journal, list your medications. Indicate any changes in dosages. If you take pain medications "as needed", keep track of how many you take every day. Keep paper and pencil near your medications and jot down the time and amount or just make hash marks. Many people like to put their daily medications in weekly pill containers available in the stores. These containers will really help you to avoid missing doses, or doubling doses accidentally.

Include a place in your journal to jot down questions for your doctor as you think of them. Then, when it is time to go to the doctor, you won't be struggling to remember what it was that you wanted to ask.

It is also helpful to look back over your journal from time to time. You may realize that you have made more progress than you thought. You may be able to identify what helped you in a previous flare–up, and to try the same thing when it happens again.

It is very therapeutic to keep this kind of journal, because once you "make your report", you are free to let go of that particular episode. Do your best to forget about all the ups and downs. If there is something you need to remember, you can go to your journal and look it up.

Have hope in the total healing that will be yours in heaven.

You will be whole, complete and pain free some day, provided you have asked Jesus to be your Lord and Savior. It is a great comfort to know that better times are ahead.

Your situation may be progressive or terminal. You may know that as bad as you feel right now, you will only feel worse in the days to come. This can be terribly depressing. God has given you the antidote for this—hope. He has given you the hope you need to see you through the worst possible circumstances. That hope is that any circumstance you face here on earth is only temporary. Not only will it end, it will be replaced by good and glorious circumstances. Your suffering on earth is incredibly short, compared to the eternity you will spend in perfect health and with wonderful circumstances in heaven. The more you suffer on earth, the more precious this hope can become for you. It is very helpful to read the Bible, looking for descriptions of what you will experience in heaven.

During the years that I have spent in continuous and sometimes extreme pain, I have found great relief in reading God's descriptions of what my future holds. Revelations 21, Isaiah 65:17-25 and Isaiah 66:10-24 provide me with pieces of the puzzle that fit together to form a picture of heaven. (Joni Eareckson Tada's book, *Heaven, Your Real Home*, has also been a great encouragement to me.)

The intriguing thing is that it seems like the pieces (the descriptions of heaven) don't fit together properly, or even that not all of the pieces are there. This is good! Think about a jigsaw puzzle. The pleasure is in working it. Once all the pieces are in place, it no longer holds your attention. You may look at the picture once in a while, but you don't spend hours with it. But since all the pieces are not in place in the puzzle of heaven, I can continue to think about them and try to fit them together in my mind. I enjoy mulling over the pieces of scripture that tell me about my future home. There is always a new piece to fit into place.

The time I spend contemplating my pain-free, blissful life to come is refreshing. As I picture myself in heaven, I begin to notice that my pain is less because my focus is on something else, something pleasant. I am rejuvenated. The afterglow of hope carries over for many hours.

Heaven doesn't mean as much to someone whose life on earth is pleasant and for whom things are the way he or she wants them, because there isn't such a great need for something better. But when life is unpleasant, the hope of heaven is very precious. It can provide you with the motivation you need to keep moving forward here on earth.

Are you certain that you have eternal life and that you will be going to heaven? It is a great blessing to be certain of your future. God's Word shows you what you need to know and do to be certain that you will spend eternity in heaven. Read the following verses. Ask God to show you His truth through them and to help you to respond to them. (Italics have been added.)

> **1 John 5:13 (NIV)** I write these things to you who believe in the name of the Son of God *so that you may know that you have eternal life.*
> **John 3:16 (Msg)** "This is how much God loved the world: He gave his Son, his one and only Son. And this is why: so that no one need be destroyed; *by believing in him, anyone can have a whole and lasting life.*
> **Romans 6:23b (NLT)** The *free gift of God is eternal life through Christ Jesus* our Lord.

The above verses indicate that you can know with certainty what your future will be. God has a plan that He wants you to participate in. Jesus made it possible for you to be *given* eternal life if you choose to believe in Him.

Romans 3:23 (NLT) For *all have sinned*; all fall short of God's glorious standard.

Ephesians 2:9 (NLT) *Salvation is not a reward for the good things we have done*, so none of us can boast about it.

Romans 6:23a (NLT) For *the wages of sin is death.*

John 14:6 Jesus answered, "*I am the way* and the truth and the life. *No one comes to the Father except through me.*

1 Peter 3:18 (NLT) Christ also suffered when he died for our sins once for all time. He never sinned, but *he died for sinners that he might bring us safely home to God.* He suffered physical death, but he was raised to life in the Spirit.

These verses show that we are all sinners. No matter how many good things you do, the fact remains–the fair reward (wage) for sin is death. You cannot overcome this fact and earn your way into heaven. God, however, paid that price for you with the death of His only son, who was without sin. This is the only payment that is sufficient to get you into heaven.

John 1:12 (NLT) But *to all who believed him and accepted him, he gave the right to become children of God.*

Ephesians 2:8 (NLT) *God saved you by his special favor when you believed.* And you can't take credit for this; it is a gift from God.

Romans 10:10 (NLT) For *it is by believing in your heart that you are made right with God, and it is by confessing with your mouth that you are saved.*

Romans 10:13 (NLT) For "Anyone who calls on the name of the Lord will be saved."

Luke 10:20 (NLT) "Rejoice because your names are registered as citizens of heaven."

God's plan for you is so simple that it is easy to overlook it. All you have to do in order to have eternal life and go to heaven is to accept God's plan. You need only to take Him at His word and believe that Jesus' death was the one and only available payment for your sins, and therefore your only possible "ticket" to heaven. (You may still question why this is so, but the necessary element is that you accept God's plan.) This can be done with a simple, heartfelt prayer like the following:

> Dear God, It is true that I don't do everything right. My thoughts, motives, and actions can be self-centered, unkind, or worse. I am a sinner. According to your word I can't earn my way to heaven no matter what I do. Thank you for allowing your only son, Jesus, who was sinless, to pay the price for my sins. I am grateful for this provision.   I do accept your plan for my salvation.   I receive Jesus into my life right now and thank you that now I have eternal life and I will go to heaven. Help me to follow you with my whole heart. In Jesus' name. Amen.

This is only the beginning of the Christian life, but it is important. It is the only way to begin it! Tell someone about your prayer. Find a Bible-based church or fellowship group that will help you to learn more about not only your eternal hope, but also about the invaluable help and hope Jesus offers you for daily living. Your decision to include Jesus in your life can make more difference in your pain journey than any other single decision you make.

Choose a starting place

This chapter has a lot of information in it to process. It would be impossible to implement all of it at once. That is not an excuse, however, for not implementing any of it! Prayerfully consider this information.   Let the Lord guide you to an attitude that you would benefit from developing more fully in your life.   Maybe one sentence or section of this chapter will stick in your mind.   (Make sure you are considering how *you* could benefit from it, not someone else.)   Talk to God about it. Talk to a friend or loved one.   Then seek to include that attitude into your life on a daily basis.

Chapter 10

The Balancing Act

*L*iving with chronic pain is like walking a tightrope. Instead of walking down a broad sidewalk as you live out your daily activities, you find yourself walking a thin line. Healthy bodies seem to adapt to periods of stress, over–exertion, or too little sleep. However, for people who live with chronic pain, some additional stress, a few nights of poor sleep, or some over-exertion can be enough to set off a significant pain flare-up. It is just like walking a tightrope; if you want to avoid a major catastrophe you will have to stay very well balanced!

Living a balanced life in the midst of your pain is indeed a balancing act. You must balance activity with rest. Carefully weigh the things you want to do against those things your body is able to do. Most of us also will have to balance the need to earn money versus the need to avoid stress. Learning to balance life with chronic pain can seem like a daunting task. But just like walking a tightrope, it can be learned. Once the skill is learned there is a real sense of accomplishment in being able to perform daily activities from such a precarious position.

Accept the reality of your pain

The first step toward mastering this balancing act is to accept the fact that you are indeed on a tightrope. In other words, admit to yourself and to those around you that chronic pain is a part of your life, that it does affect your activities, and that you are going to be living with it for the foreseeable future.

When you refuse to accept the reality of your pain, your pain levels generally go up because you do things that aggravate your problem. Then you either experience another flare-up, have a major health crash, find yourself having to cancel important activities due to elevated pain levels, use up your monthly pain medication way too soon, or (at the very least) become cranky and hard to live with. This is rather like walking on a tightrope and falling off—you hurt yourself and you may also hurt whoever is around you. Any way you look at it, when you behave as if you are still walking on solid ground when in reality you are on a tightrope, a price will be paid.

Once you accept the fact that, like it or not, you are walking through life on the tightrope of chronic pain, you can begin to work on improving your balance and on avoiding some of the crashes and falls you may have previously experienced. There are many useful and effective techniques for balancing life with chronic pain. It is quite an adventure to perfect them.

Note: There is a time to search for an end to your pain, and there is also a time to move beyond that search and to work on maximizing your life in the midst of your pain. If a doctor (or two) that you have reason to trust is quite certain that there is no reasonable way to end your pain, then it is most probably time to stop searching for a cure and to start looking for ways to reduce your pain instead. The act of making that decision and changing your focus should already reduce your pain somewhat. When you are looking for a cure, it is very common to focus on how bad you feel (and therefore how much you need the cure), rather than focusing on how you can minimize your pain.

Listen to your body and respond to its message

The best starting place for learning to balance your life with chronic pain is simply to pay attention to what you do each day and how it affects your body. Hopefully, you have started a health journal by now. Include in your entries your activities during the day, how you felt while you were doing them, and how you felt afterwards. When your pain levels are up, think back over the day and note what you did. When your levels are down, do the same. Ask God to guide your thoughts and to help you to notice the things that matter for your situation.

Many years ago, shortly after my journey with pain began, I was inventorying my activities and how they increased or decreased my pain levels. I discovered that the single biggest pain amplifier in my daily activities was driving or riding in a car. It took many more years to get a handle on *why* this was so, but even without knowing why, I reduced my pain by finding ways to combine errands, thus spending less time in the car. Eventually I switched to a car with a smoother ride and an automatic transmission, which helped my pain levels even more.

It was also obvious that I got worse as the day went on. Lying down during the day made it possible for me to do things after dinner. Otherwise I was in too much pain to move. In no way did these discoveries end my pain, but they did give me some control over it. I was beginning to manage my pain—to have some power over it—instead of just feeling like it was controlling me.

Your body can give you very important information that even your doctor would be hard-pressed to discover. The trick is to not get bogged down in every ache and pain, but instead, to learn to observe, make notes, and go on with your day. Then pick a time to carefully and prayerfully consider your journal. Look for trends. Ask God to show you what you need to see. Make some adjustments according to your observations and see what happens.

Be on the same team as your body

An essential element of the process of balancing life with chronic pain is learning to work with your body instead of fighting it. It is common to take a strong, healthy body for granted. You expect to be able to do most anything you really want to (within reason). When, for some reason, your body no longer functions as well as it used to, you may push it to its limits, trying to force it to perform as you think it should. This is one example of fighting your body. It is as if you were on one team and your body was on the opposing team.

Resist the temptation to fight your body and aim instead to see the bigger picture. Admit the fact that you aren't a superhero. You can and should quit an activity, even right in the middle of it, if your body is telling you to quit (in other words, if your pain is escalating.) You hurt yourself and those around you when you keep pushing until you cause a flare-up in your pain. Your ability to live out the rest of your daily activities is reduced and you set off a roller coaster effect, one where the physical, mental, emotional, and financial side-effects all come, along with the pain flare-up. It just isn't worth that price to try to keep going when your body is telling you that you shouldn't. (If you are an athlete who is used to pushing through pain to train or compete, this may be a foreign idea to you. Remember, chronic pain requires a different approach than acute pain.)

It is okay to get mad at your body because it annoys, disappoints, or hurts you, but stay on the same team with it. It's the only body you will have until you get to heaven, so it will be to your advantage to work with it rather than working against it. Take some time to express your anger at your pain and how it interferes with your life. Then thank God for the perfect body that is waiting for you in heaven and move on with your plan for keeping your present body as functional as possible. Performing your daily activities on a tightrope is challenge enough; being engaged in a duel with your body at the same time will complicate things unnecessarily.

Another important way to work with your body is to be careful about how you "feed" it pain medication. It seems pretty reasonable to take your pain medication only when your pain is high, when you feel you really need it. At first glance, this appears to be a good way to keep from taking too much pain medication. However, this is not the case. When your pain is soaring, it takes a lot more medication to get it down to a tolerable level than it would have taken to keep it at a tolerable level.

Keeping your base pain level down by taking your pain medication on a schedule will help your body to cope with your pain more successfully. It reduces the wear and tear on your body caused by spikes in pain. These spikes increase muscle tension levels, excite your nerves, and set off other pain-producing problems. Taking your medication on schedule helps also to keep inflammation, muscle tension, and overall tissue irritability down. It may be helpful to increase a medication before a certain activity to help prevent pain flares, but as rule, stick to your schedule.

Chapter 11

Pacing

$\mathscr{P}$acing involves learning your body's limits and timing your activities in such a way that you don't exceed those limits. Learning to pace yourself is a huge issue when balancing life with chronic pain. The pace you kept on "flat ground" (life without pain) just doesn't work on a tightrope.

Simply put, pacing means choosing your daily activities and the length of time spent doing them in such a way that your pain levels aren't elevated by what you do. This does not mean stopping your activities because you hurt; you may always hurt. It means adjusting your activities to avoid *major increases* in the amount that you hurt.

Pacing involves two main elements–the activities you choose to do in a day, and the length of time you spend on each activity. The goal is to find the combination of these elements that allow you to be as active as possible day after day and week after week. You are looking for a pace that you can *sustain*, rather than doing so much on one day that it interferes with your ability to do things on the next day. In other words, you are trying to stay on the tightrope all the way from one end to the other, instead of falling off part way across it.

Many people never find this pace. Their lives consist of a series of mad dashes, trying to make it across the tightrope without falling off. Rarely do they succeed. Instead they fall off and injure themselves. Then, as soon as they can, they hop back on again, only to dash a short distance before falling once again.

In order to develop the balance required to make it from one end of the tightrope to the other, it is necessary to slow down and work on balancing skills, rather than focusing only on the activity you want to accomplish while crossing the tightrope. When your balancing skills are well developed, you will find that you can move quite quickly from one end of the tightrope to the other without falling off. *Pacing is the primary skill required for your balancing act.*

In order to live successfully with chronic pain, it is absolutely vital that you slow down and find the pace at which your body can function without aggravating your problems. This allows your body to turn its attention to restoring and healing itself, rather than needing to attempt to recover from a continual series of traumas. You will find that reducing the frequency of pain spikes and flare-ups will reduce the stress level your body is under, and that pacing has actually lowered your pain level. Once you have stabilized your pain, you can try to carefully add activities one by one to see how much you can do without aggravating it again.

Setting a pace

Keep track of how long you can do various activities before your pain level increases. Check your health journal for useful information and take additional notes as needed. Write down your "safe" length of time. Then, use a timer to stop yourself several minutes *before* you hit your time limit. (This will require discipline. I finally had to get an obnoxious-sounding timer that didn't stop screaming until it was manually turned off. I placed it on the other side of the room so that I had to stop what I was doing in order to get up and turn it off!) When your time is up, take a break. You may want to practice some deep breathing to help your body to relax, or perhaps do a few stretches. Change to another activity or rest if you need to. Repeat this process with your various activities throughout the day.

Because I had a long attention span and a strong drive to complete any project I began, I completely rejected this approach when it was first presented to me. I was accustomed to sticking with a project until I was in tears with pain, or until I hurt so much that I simply couldn't function. Generally it took an hour or less for me to get to this point any way, so I had no desire to quit any sooner than that.

However, my pain was steadily increasing. Day after day went by without me even feeling well enough to start a project. My misery made me became more willing to change my ways. I tried doing an activity for a short time, quitting before my pain level went up. I found only one disadvantage, but several advantages to this procedure. The disadvantage was that I didn't finish the project that day, but the advantages were many:

- My mood improved because I had done something to get my mind off my pain.
- I managed to do something without increasing my pain level. (This was practically unheard of for me at the time.)
- I was able to do more short sessions of the same activity later that day and on the following days.
- Within several days I had finished the project! (This was something that I had rarely managed to do, even when I pushed myself to extreme pain levels.)

I had found a pace that I could maintain. Compared to what I used to accomplish before I lived with chronic pain, it was pathetic, but I was learning that it was pointless to compare myself to former times. I was learning to walk a tightrope and I had finally made it from one end to the other without falling off. By limiting the amount of time I spent on an activity at any one time, I actually increased the total amount of time that I was able to perform that activity.

Note: Distraction is a real friend to all of us who live with pain. Simply getting involved in a conversation or activity can distract your mind from the pain messages it is receiving. You may hardly notice your pain for hours. It provides a wonderful break from the tyranny of pain.

Warning: It is also possible to be so distracted from your pain that you don't notice how it has been elevating. Although you may be enjoying yourself at the moment, too much distraction is an enemy rather than a friend if you have allowed it to lead you beyond your reasonable limits. Be sure to check in with your body every so often and to respond to what it is telling you, even if you are currently being distracted from your pain.

Improving your Pacing–select your activities with your pain index in mind

You may find that there are activities that increase your pain level the moment you start doing them. There does not seem to be any "safe" length of time for you to do these activities. Yet they may be very important parts of your day. This brings us to the second element of pacing–carefully choosing your activities. Choosing what will and won't get done in a day is challenging enough, even without chronic pain. You have to carefully balance work-related activities, recreational activities, family and social activities, and outreach activities (acts of kindness that are an expression of your love for God). Weigh all these against your available time, energy, and resources. Naturally, there always seems to be more to do than time, energy, and money allows.

Pacing involves adding one more factor to this priority system, *your pain index*. Whether you are aware of it or not, you have probably already developed some system for prioritizing your activities. *Your pain index is the social, occupational, spiritual, or recreational benefits of an activity, compared to how it affects your pain level.* If that activity is beneficial at both ends, it has a low pain index, and is therefore a good choice. If doing that activity is necessary but is very detrimental to your pain level, then the score for it falls towards the mid–range of your index. That activity must be carefully considered for ways to either adjust or even replace it. If an activity scores high on pain and is anything less than essential, it gets a high pain index score. It would be best to completely avoid that particular activity for now.

It may seem awkward at first to incorporate your pain index into your priority system for choosing activities. Often you do things "because they need to be done". You may not think about how they affect you. But if an activity greatly increases your pain level, someone else may need to do that activity for you, or it may need to be done in a modified way. In the end it may cost less to hire the job out than to pay the medical bills that result from continuing to do the activity. (In my case, scrubbing and vacuuming greatly increased my pain levels. My husband graciously agreed to do many of the household chores.)

Look closely to see which ones are the activities that flare your pain. Regardless of whether or not you are presently willing to modify or quit any of your activities, it will help you to recognize how much effect they have on you. Here are some questions to begin evaluating your activities with regard to your pain index:

• *Does this activity increase my pain level? How much? Can it be adjusted? (Can it be done in shorter segments, done more ergonomically, or done in some other way that is not as hard on my body?)*

- *If I can't adapt the activity, can it be replaced by another activity that doesn't increase my pain (or at least, one that doesn't increase it as much?)*
- *Is it essential that I do this activity? Could someone else do this activity, allowing me to do something else in exchange that doesn't flare my pain as much?*
- *What can I do today and still feel good? (That is, as good as I ever feel, which is far better than the worst I feel.)*
- *Would the rest of my week be better if I didn't do this activity? Be honest: are your pain levels higher for a few days after each time you do this? If they are, but you still really don't want to give the activity up, plan for the recuperation time you will need afterwards. This will help to minimize your damage.*

Any reductions you can make in the things that flare your pain will help you. Start with the easier ones. Pray about the harder issues, such as vocation related activities or favorite activities that flare your pain significantly. Ultimately, you may want to change or restructure these, but before that is accomplished there are other, more simple changes that can still help you a lot.

Small changes to things that you do repeatedly can make a big difference. This could include things like:

- *Use a headset with your phone instead of holding it between your shoulder and ear.*
- *Replace your work, running, or walking shoes with ones that give you better support.*
- *Improve the ergonomics of your workspace.*
- *Get a better mattress for your bed.*
- *Avoid sitting on your wallet. Carry it in your front pocket instead.*
- *Avoid carrying your purse on your shoulder. Carry it under your arm or use a fanny pack. (Or at least lighten the load in it.)*

A good physical or occupational therapist will have a wealth of information about small changes that can make significant differences in your pain level. Ask your doctor to give you a referral. Take your list of activities, including how they affect your pain levels, with you to your appointment.

An opportunity for new activities

It is reasonable to assume that, as your body develops new requirements due to pain, you may benefit by finding some new activities that will better match your present circumstances. This could include anything from new family outings to new hobbies or a new vocation. It is not always easy to give up an activity. However, try giving up an activity for a month. If it reduces your pain levels significantly, the reduction in pain may motivate you to fill its place in your life with something else.

In my case, I had already removed many activities out of my life in order to make it possible for me to lie down and relax my muscles frequently throughout the day, as this was the only real relief I found from my pain. Medications and a wide variety of therapies had yet to provide much help. I had decreased my activities outside of the home to doctor's appointments, Sunday church, grocery shopping (with someone to help me), and my two favorite activities–directing a youth handbell choir and playing in an adult handbell choir. My medical team had encouraged me not to give up these favorite activities so that I would have something to look forward to in my routine.

But within a few months I was no longer enjoying handbells. My pain levels were so high while playing or directing that I could barely focus on what I was doing, much less enjoy it. It would take three or four days for my pain to go back down after a rehearsal. Finally I decided to take a month off from both handbell groups, just to see how that affected my health. It turned out to be a wonderful relief not to have the pain flare so violently a couple of times each week.

As much as I loved those activities and especially the people I shared them with, it was clear to me that I needed to give up handbells, at least until my health situation changed. This was a very difficult decision for me. I had invested hours of my time in arranging the music the youth choir performed, and I was also very involved in the lives of the kids. Bells were a big part of my life. It felt like a real defeat to surrender these activities, yet it was senseless to put myself through the extra pain they produced.

Shortly after making the decision to quit bells, an opportunity came up to help with the costumes in the drama department at my son's school. Soon, while one son was acting and our other son (and sometimes also my husband) worked on set construction, I was helping with costumes. Saying 'no' to one activity had paved the way for me to get involved in a different one that proved to be equally as rewarding, and far less aggravating to my pain.

As I look back on those years, I am very thankful that God provided that opportunity for our family to do something together before our sons went their separate ways for college. I am quite sure that I would have been too busy with my other activities to have helped with costumes if pain hadn't redirected my life. I thank God for this change and for many other changes in my life that my pain has necessitated. I am a better person for them.

Conserve your energy, plan your day

Another way to improve your balance while living with chronic pain is to learn to conserve your energy. Avoid overfilling your day. Decide what is most necessary or important to do each day (include something enjoyable), and plan your day around those things. Your day will proceed much better if you make these decisions before the day gets going, rather than during the day. It is hard to opt out of a desirable activity just when it is right in front of you. But it is easier to say no if you have made your choices ahead of time, and you know that you are passing on one activity so that you can do another one of a higher priority.

If you know you have a strenuous day coming up, try to plan an easy day before and after it. This will help you to have the energy you need for the strenuous day, and will also give you some time to recover afterward. Planning for heavy days in this way may allow you to perform activities that elevate your pain levels without causing a significant flare-up.

Choosing your activities wisely means not only weighing how the activity affects your pain level against how necessary it is or how much satisfaction it gives you. It also means realistically assessing how much you can do in one day, and carefully filling your schedule with the higher priority items. Your wise choices reduce your pain level by avoiding pain-producing activities. You have also avoided the pain-producing stress that is a result of an over-full schedule.

Expect to make time for your pain

When chronic pain is an element in your life, it is like adding another member to your household. It affects routines and requires attention. If it is ignored and not attended to, it will create havoc. Given the appropriate time and attention, it will fit much more smoothly into your life.

We have looked at ways to make time for your pain by resting when your pain rises, or by planning a lighter schedule to keep stress and fatigue to a minimum. There are other proactive ways to take time for your pain that will pay good dividends. Take the time to eat nutritious meals, to focus on relaxing your body, to get appropriate exercise and adequate sleep. Chronic pain can actually encourage the development of healthy habits because the reward of less pain provides a powerful incentive to make some changes.

You may get significant benefits from investing even a small amount of time. Two minutes spent on stretching or loosening up exercises, done faithfully two or three times throughout your day, may be enough to keep your muscles from tightening up and increasing your pain. You can reduce pain by taking time to prepare or purchase food that gives your body the building blocks it needs to restore itself. Working time into your schedule for 30 minutes of walking or some other exercise may give you not only energy that you haven't had for a long time, it can also reduce your pain. In the end you will get your 30 minutes back plus more, because exercise generally helps you to feel better, allowing you to be more active. (Talk to your doctor before starting a new exercise program to be sure that you choose one that is appropriate for you.)

You have just read about several things you can do to balance your life as you live with chronic pain. In all honesty, these are very healthy and helpful skills that will benefit anyone, whether or not you have chronic pain. But for those who walk the tightrope of chronic pain, these skills can make all the difference between successfully and gracefully traversing the tightrope, or repeatedly falling to the ground. Believe it or not, your life can be happy and fulfilling with chronic pain. Balancing your life and pacing wisely are vital ingredients in achieving success.

Chapter 12

Healthy Habits: Nutrition

Healthy habits promote a healthy body. The healthier your body is, the more capable it will be of healing itself and of neutralizing or minimizing pain. Whether or not you are the "picture of fitness", it is certainly to your advantage to do everything you can to promote wellness in your body. Wellness is not a simply a lack of symptoms. It is a state of balance and wellbeing. Wellness is attained by supplying your body with its basic needs, such as good nutrition, sleep, relaxation, and exercise.

Our society is struggling with increasing percentages of people developing serious health problems, such as diabetes, cancer, heart disease, or obesity, at much younger ages than in previous generations. As researchers are looking for the best ways to reverse this trend, time after time they have come up with the same answer—a healthy diet, exercise, and sufficient sleep to reduce the risk of acquiring these health problems and/or reducing their severity. In this technological age, people tend to expect high-tech solutions to their health and pain problems. But fancy drugs will not satisfy your body's basic needs as much as the simple and healthy habits of eating right, exercising, and getting sufficient relaxation and sleep will.

Avoid Popping Pills

Americans have come to expect pills to maintain and restore their health. If you expect pills to solve your problems or make you feel better, whenever you don't feel good you usually will take a pill to remedy the situation. A healthier habit would be to listen to your body's complaints and to make adjustments to reduce them. For example, a tension headache can be helped by changing positions, stretching or walking a bit, massaging your scalp, and doing some deep breathing exercises to relax, instead of reaching for a bottle of pills. As a preventative measure, it is wise to schedule a few minutes several times a day to do these simple exercises.

If you are on a lot of medications, it is possible that you would actually feel better if you reduced the number you take. They all have side effects and interact with each other to some degree. Discuss this with your doctor or pharmacist. But first do your homework. List each medication you take, why you are taking it, and how you take it (as needed or on a schedule.) If you don't know what a medication is for, find out. You can look each drug up on the Internet (*www.drugs.com*) and see what condition it treats, what are its side effects, and how it interacts with other drugs. Then request some time to talk to your doctor. Bring the list and see if there are duplications, or some that you could try doing without. It is usually best to change only one drug at a time so you can tell how your body is affected by the change.

Nutrition

For most of human history people ate what was grown and available right around them. Commodities like sugar, salt, and chocolate were expensive and not readily available in many areas. Meals were largely the same day after day because they consisted of the food that was available in that area at that time of year. Desserts and sweets were occasional treats. Portions of food were limited because the available food was limited.

What a different scenario that is from today's all-you-can-eat buffets and fast food restaurants with super-sized menu items! In our present society we have virtually limitless types of food available to us, and yet the food we eat is, for the most part, less nutritious than what our ancestors ate.   Why? Because we tend to eat a lot of quick, convenience foods that are prepackaged and processed. You may not even be aware that you have been exchanging nutrition for convenience.

In the past, food was eaten when and if it was available, to appease hunger and provide nourishment for energy.   As food has become more available, people tend to eat not just to reduce hunger, but also for emotional reasons–because the food appeals to them, as a reward, or as a social activity.   Check yourself. What are the main reasons that you open your mouth and insert food? Significant hunger? The nutritional value of the food? Social reasons (going out with friends or family), or emotional reasons (I feel like it, I need something to give me a boost)?.

The food you put into your mouth affects your wellbeing much more than most of us realize. In reality, eating is your body's only opportunity to get the raw ingredients it needs to give you energy to be active, to build and repair its cells, and to fight off any illnesses or invasions. You can reduce your pain levels and improve your quality of life by thoughtfully choosing what you eat. Here are some interesting facts about nutrition and wellness:

- **_Diet can reduce back pain._**
  "The omega-3 fatty acids in fish oil seem to help some back pain sufferers to do away with prescription non steroidal anti-inflammatory drugs (NSAIDS).   In a study of 125 people taking NSAIDS for non-surgical neck and back pain, 59 percent reported discontinuing their NSAIDS after less than three months of taking between 1.2 and 2.4 grams of fish-oil

supplements containing the omega-3 fatty acids EPA and DHA. Sixty percent stated that their overall pain and joint pain had improved." (Surgical Neurology, April 2006)

- *Diet can reduce pain by reducing inflammation.*
  "Emphasizing foods high in antioxidants, such as fruits and vegetables, will reduce inflammation and its related symptoms. Some studies of fish oil, nuts, and various fruits and vegetables show a reduction in inflammatory markers and symptoms of heart disease, diabetes, rheumatoid arthritis, osteoarthritis, gout, and some inflammatory bowel disorders."

- *Diet can boost or decrease your immune system.*
  "The food choices you make and the nutrients supplied by your diet can either strengthen your immune system so that it protects you from illness and help you recover sooner if you get sick, or they can weaken your body's defenses, leaving you vulnerable to everything that's going around." (Dr. Andrew Weil's Self Healing, December 2005)

- *Diet is a major factor in cancer.*
  "An estimated 35 to 60 percent of all cancers are linked to dietary factors. (Dr. Andrew Weil's Self Healing, June 2006)

- *Nutrition effects our life span.*
  "In research that spanned nine European countries and included more than 74,000 healthy men and women aged 60 and over, people who closely followed the typical Mediterranean eating plan – which emphasizes

fresh fruits and vegetables, whole grains, beans, nuts, fish, and olive oil, and contains less meat, poultry, and dairy products and moderate amounts of alcohol – enjoyed greater longevity over a seven-year period." (British Medical Journal, April 8, 2005)

There is much you can do to improve your health as you sit down to eat each day. This is good news! You need to eat every day, so why not improve your health as you do it? The eating plans mentioned above–the Mediterranean diet and the anti-inflammatory diet–are very similar. The Mayo Clinic describes an anti-inflammatory diet as follows:

"An anti-inflammatory diet focuses on increased consumption of vegetable proteins such as legumes, fruits, vegetables, whole grains, and certain types of fats. This means a limited intake of meat, dairy, sweets, and refined and processed foods, although an occasional piece of dark chocolate may help satisfy a sweet tooth. Water and green tea are also recommended." (Mayo Clinic Women's HealthSource, November 2005)

If inflammation is a major source of your pain, you will benefit from learning more about the anti-inflammatory eating plan. By adjusting the fats you eat and a few other foods, you should enjoy a noticeable reduction in your pain levels. The Mayo Clinic is one good source of information. They will mail you literature or you can access them at *www.MayoClinic.org*.

If depression, low energy levels, and mood swings contribute to your pain problem, you may be able to improve your situation considerably by adjusting the kinds of carbohydrates and the amount of sugar you consume.

"Eating a carbohydrate-rich snack or meal can help you feel more relaxed by increasing levels of the neurotransmitter *serotonin*. But more refined carbs, such as products made with flour and sugar, also cause blood-sugar levels to rise rapidly and then fall steeply. This roller-coaster effect can lead to overeating, weight gain, and insulin resistance in genetically susceptible people. You're better off by choosing less refined carbs like whole grains and beans, and starchy vegetables like sweet potatoes and winter squash, which can raise serotonin levels without the unhealthy swings in blood sugar." (Dr. Andrew Weil's Self Healing, June 2004)

Don't give up if your present eating habits are not much like the ones described in these eating plans. You have the most to gain by developing some healthy habits. Pick one habit to adjust–increase the fruit and vegetables you eat each day, or reduce your sweets or the unhealthy fats you eat.

You may want to use the "plate plan" in order to avoid *empty calories*. You may notice that many of the foods you regularly eat don't fit into any of these categories–French fries, sweets, chips, dips, and sauces. These foods are empty calories: they don't provide your body with significant nutrition, yet they may have plenty of calories. At each mealtime, aim to fill half of your plate with fruits and vegetables, another fourth with healthy grains, and the last fourth with protein foods. Put nutritious foods on your plate first. After you have eaten, then put a limited amount of "empty calorie" food on your plate. (If you start eating with empty calories, your appetite may be satisfied before your body has received the nutrients it needs.) It is always a good idea to put your food on your plate rather than "grazing" from a bowl or box. You will have better control of your portions this way.

Be alert for mental pitfalls associated with eating. Retrain yourself to recognize that the main purpose of eating is to provide your body with the nutrients it needs to feel good and function well, not to enjoy your favorite goodies or to relieve stress. Eat for the sake of your body, not for emotional or social reasons. The best way to deal with anxiety and stress is not by eating. Go for a walk, practice relaxation techniques, call a friend, watch a movie, pray, or read your Bible. God's Word is a powerful antidote for stress and emotional struggles.

Just like counting to ten before saying anything when you are mad, if you think about why you are heading for food before you put a bite in your mouth, you may be able to significantly improve your mood, your health, and your immune system. Recognize the power you have to control your health. Remember that you are feeding your body, not just your appetite, with the food you put in your mouth. Your body will show its appreciation by its increased wellness!

Chapter 13

Exercise, Relaxation and Sleep

Exercise

Our bodies not only have nutritional needs, they also require exercise to maintain wellness. Just as cars suffer when they sit for too long without being run, our muscles, joints, and bones need regular activity to keep them healthy and strong.

In today's world, machines deprive you of much of the exercise your ancestors got as a part of daily living, so you must make a conscious effort to give your body the exercise it needs. This is especially important for people with chronic pain. It is natural to think that if you hurt you need to cut back on your activity level. For acute pain problems like sprains and other injuries it may help to limit your activity, but chronic pain tends to improve with consistent, appropriate activity.

Pain and the conditions causing it may limit the activities you are able to do, but it will be well worth your while to search until you find something you can do and to make it a part of your daily routine. Exercise can be just as important for your body as the prescription medications you take. Here are some interesting facts about exercise and pain.

- ***Regular exercise prolongs life expectancy, and improves health conditions***
  "Researchers Against Inactivity-related Diseases, a new advocacy group, has coined the

term Sedentary Death Syndrome (SeDS) to refer to the 250,000 or more deaths each year it says could be prevented by engaging in regular exercise. It also claims that 35 health problems, from obesity to depression, are caused or worsened by a lack of exercise. Just as inactivity can cause or worsen many health conditions, regular exercise can also *improve* them. In fact, a recent review of published research confirms that moderate physical activity on most days of the week is associated with up to a 30% reduced risk of dying from *all* causes (Medicine and Science in Sports and Exercise, June 2001).

- *Physical activity reduces pain*
  "Physical activity can help reduce chronic pain by prompting your body to release *endorphins*, natural pain-relieving chemicals. Regular exercise also gives you more energy to cope with your pain, and helps alleviate anxiety and depression, which can make pain more difficult to manage. The key is balance — exercising too much or too intensely can make pain worse, while moderate, consistent physical activity helps." (Mayo Clinic Women's HealthSource Special Report November 2005)

- *Exercise improves mood*
  "Regular physical activity appears to boost mood and keep your brain young, fit, and sharp. Moving your body may also work its magic on your mind by improving the flow of oxygen-rich blood to the brain; by increasing body temperature, which relaxes tense muscles; by reducing levels of *cortisol*, a stress hormone that's directly toxic to brain cells; and by increasing

the connections between brain neurons that sharpen memory.

There is solid evidence that physical activity is highly effective for treating mild-to-moderate depression and is of benefit in severe cases as well...Studies show that aerobic activity done at moderate intensity for at least 20 minutes about three times a week seems to lessen anxious thoughts." (Dr. Andrew Weil's Self Healing December 2005)

• *The "exercise prescription"*

"What natural remedy helps lower blood pressure, ease arthritis pain, and boost energy? A brisk 30-to 45- minute walk, at least five days a week. I suggest patients take this prescription for 'lifestyle medicine' as seriously as they do medications and supplements." (Dr. Andrew Weil's Self Healing, September 2001)

Muscles that aren't used weaken quickly. When they are weak they don't support the bones and joints as well. This increases susceptibility to joint injuries and bone fractures. Also if muscles become too weak to adequately do their job, other muscles have to help out. If they weren't designed for that job, they will fatigue quickly, spasm, and create more pain.

Personally, I have found that the best way for me to reduce the multitude of aches and pains I wake up with daily (actually *they* generally wake *me* up), is to get up, get dressed, and go for a walk. There were times when I could only walk a half mile or less due to my extreme pain. But even when my pain was the worst, the motivation that got me up and going was thinking about how much better I would feel after my walk. When I don't start my day with a walk I can always tell, because my pain levels are up.

Three categories of exercise

The three categories of exercise your body needs are *aerobic, flexibility and balance, and strength training.* By planning to include moderate amounts of each kind of exercise in your weekly routine, you will minimize your risk of falls, fractures and injuries, reduce your pain, and improve your mood and energy levels.

Aerobic exercise includes activities such as walking, swimming, biking, dancing, gardening, and other activities that increase oxygen intake and heart rate.

Flexibility and balance exercises help reduce joint stiffness and prevent muscles from shortening and tightening through regular, gentle stretching. This makes movement easier and less painful. Yoga, Pilates, and Tai Chi are popular ways to do flexibility and balance training. Your physical therapist or other trained professional can also give you simple exercises to do at home. It is especially important to stretch and strengthen the core muscles deep in your midsection that affect your posture and support the spine. When these muscles are weak, back or neck pain frequently develops because other muscles are overworking to compensate for core muscle weakness.

Strength training with light weights is the third part of an exercise plan. The idea is not to become "muscle men or women", but just to prevent the muscle loss and fat gain that naturally occur with age. Stronger muscles help to protect joints by creating a natural "brace" that supports them. Strong leg muscles can help to brace a troublesome knee. Strong back and abdominal muscles support your low back, reducing back pain.

It is recommended that you get 30-45 minutes of aerobic activity at least five days a week, strength training two or three times a week (which can be aerobic, depending on what you do), and flexibility and balance training several times a week. Portions of the latter can be done in front of the TV.

Before beginning new exercises, talk to your doctor or physical therapist to see what limitations or guidelines he or she recommends for you. Then you may want to work with your physical therapist, a personal trainer, or some other qualified professional who can assess your situation, give you an exercise plan, and make sure it is working well for you. Once you have your doctor's approval, you can begin by simply being more active.

Aim to increase your activity by five minutes a day every couple of weeks until you are active for 30-45 minutes a day, most days of the week. 30-45 minutes of brisk activity most days of the week is the minimum recommendation for wellness. This is *total minutes per day*. It doesn't have to be done all at once. If you are presently very inactive, start by just trying to take the "long way" of doing things instead of the shortest way. This means doing things like walking through all the rooms of the house on your way to the bathroom, or walking to your neighbor's mailbox before returning to yours to get your mail. Use stairs instead of the elevator if you can. When shopping in a store, once you have made your selections, take a lap around the store before checking out. Try doing a stretching routine while you watch TV.

Set aside a daily time to exercise. Pick a form of exercise that appeals to you. Get an appropriate exercise video and follow along in your living room, walk with a friend, mall walk, listen to your favorite music while you exercise, or play with your children or grandchildren. Rotate between different activities. Just be faithful and stick with your plan.

Relaxation

Just as bodies are designed to exercise, they are also designed to benefit from regular relaxation. This is more than just sitting down to watch a TV show or movie. Relaxation means actively decreasing tension in your body and mind.

There are many ways to practice relaxation. For instance, deep breathing is a simple and effective relaxation technique. Other relaxation techniques include meditation, yoga, guided imagery, biofeedback, and self-hypnosis.

When you relax, your heart rate and blood pressure go down. This increases the flow of blood to your major muscles and reduces muscle tension. This in turn will reduce your pain levels. Relaxation is one more tool available to you that can reduce your pain without cost or side effects.

You may want to try yoga or some kind of meditation. When you focus your mind on something peaceful--tuning out pressures and distractions--your body benefits. This is why meditation is called a "mind-body" process. When the mind is focused it slows down and calms, which allows the body to relax. Both mind and body are favorably affected.

My favorite form of meditation is sitting comfortably in the swing in our backyard, listening to the birds, and focusing my mind on a short Bible verse as I practice deep breathing. I enjoy the present moment, soaking up its beauty as I feel the sunshine and the breeze. My mind is kept from wandering as I simply focus on the goodness of God, His love, His faithfulness, or what ever the Bible verse might be about. Five minutes spent like this leaves me more rested than a half hour nap. (Brain waves actually change during meditation–it is affecting your body as well as your mind.)

Probably the simplest form of relaxation is *deep breathing*. Most adults breathe from their chests. Deep breathing is when you *breathe from your diaphragm*. Try sitting comfortably with your feet flat on the floor or lying down on your back. Inhale slowly through your nose. As your lungs fill with air, let your lower abdomen relax and expand too. (It may help to put a hand on your abdomen). When your lungs are full and your lower abdomen has expanded, slowly let the air out through your mouth. Repeat this, allowing your body to relax more with each breath. Focus your mind on your breathing to keep it from thinking about your to-do list or on other distractions. This will allow your mind to relax as well as your body.

Three or four minutes of deep breathing can calm and refresh you, reducing your anxiety and pain, improving your sleep, and relieving muscle tension. When pain or tension are on the rise, take a few minutes to practice some deep breathing. Aim for at least 3 to 5 deep breathing sessions each day. Traffic jams, doctors appointments, and other stressful moments are great opportunities to enjoy the benefits of relaxation through deep breathing.

Sleep

Sleep is not the passive state you may imagine. It is a complex series of stages, each with significant changes in your muscle activity, brain waves, eye movement, respiration and heart rate. For example, during the deep (delta) sleep stage, your muscles are completely relaxed and your blood pressure, pulse, and respiration decrease. Your body produces increased amounts of immune system modulators which boost your natural immunities. This, along with an increase in the secretion of a growth hormone, allows your body a good opportunity to grow and repair cells.

So while you sleep, your body is being restored, rejuvenated, and energized. At the same time, gastrointestinal, cardiovascular and immune functions are regulated, and the brain reorganizes and categorizes information. Sleep is not a time of inactivity! These are only a few of the activities that take place each night as you sleep. Sleep is a critical piece of the puzzle of good health.

There are, however, an estimated 50 to 70 percent of people with chronic pain who suffer from disturbed sleep. This means that all these processes don't have time to complete their work. This further complicates pain problems.

There are many factors that contribute to sleep problems. Pain makes it difficult to fall asleep and stay asleep because you notice your pain more when you lie still in bed compared to when you are engaged in activities that provide distraction. It can be impossible to get comfortable. Besides that, chronic pain depletes serotonin, the "feel good" neurotransmitter, which is also essential for sleep. Daily exercise promotes good sleep, but people with chronic pain often don't feel good enough to exercise. Many medications have side effects that interfere with sleep too.

Since sleep directly affects your energy, mood, alertness, memory, body weight, productivity, creativity, and good health, it's easy to see that you need good sleep. Let's look at how you can improve the quality of your sleep. Here are some ideas to consider:

Routine

Have a routine. Go to bed at the same time each night and get up at the same time each morning. Use the last hour before bedtime to prepare for sleep. Begin to unwind and relax. Write down things that are on your mind–unfinished jobs, plans for the next day, concerns, and worries. Take a few minutes to pray about them. Then leave them with God and turn your mind to restful, relaxing things. This is a good time to practice relaxation techniques. Many people use this time for reading. Read until you are sleepy and then get into bed and turn out the lights.

Food consumption

Avoid eating within 3 hours of bedtime If possible, eat heavy meals at midday, and light meals in the evening. Avoid foods that cause heartburn or indigestion. If you need to settle your stomach, have a small snack that is high in carbohydrates and low in protein. Avoid caffeine (including chocolate) and alcohol and limit or eliminate nicotine.

Warm bath

A warm bath before bedtime sends blood away from the brain and makes you feel drowsy. The lowering of your body temperature after the bath will initiate sleepiness. Regular exercise also enhances sleep, but make sure not to exercise near bedtime.

Surroundings

Check your surroundings to be sure they are conducive to good sleep. Is your bed comfortable? Does it provide good support? The best way to check this is to go to a store and spend several minutes lying on their beds. If you find that the store's beds are significantly more comfortable than yours, it may be time for a new bed.

Your pillow is important too. Your spine needs to be well supported from your skull to your tailbone. An extra pillow between your knees (if you sleep on your side), or under them (if you sleep on your back), will help you maintain a good sleeping posture. If you work with a physical or occupational therapist, have them help you develop a good setup for sleeping.

Make sure that your bedroom is dark and a comfortable temperature (cool is more restful than too warm.) Get curtains or shades that keep outside light out. Not only your eyes, but also your skin, sense the presence of light and will affect the quality of your sleep.

When you can't fall asleep

If you can't fall asleep, get out of bed and read awhile or do light housework until you become sleepy. Spending too much time in bed, especially when you are not sleeping, makes it even harder to sleep. Limit daytime naps to 30 minutes if you are having trouble falling asleep at night. Trying to fall asleep frequently makes it all the harder to sleep. Generally it is better to unwind and to do relaxing and restful things until you become sleepy, rather than focusing on trying to get to sleep.

If you have trouble turning off your mind enough to drift off to sleep, try listening to peaceful music or background sounds. My favorite is to listen to dramatized versions of the Bible on CD. It's important to have a CD player that turns off automatically.

Work with your medical professionals to maximize bedtime restfulness. If pain keeps you awake, other than the things mentioned above, it may also be possible to adjust medication dosages and timing to reduce your awareness of pain. You may be able to take your last 2 doses of medication closer together, rather than spacing them evenly throughout the day, to help you be drowsy at bedtime.

It is also possible that a medication you are taking is interfering with your sleep. Read the information that comes with your prescription or check on the Internet. If insomnia, excitability, or agitation are possible side effects, try taking that medication as far from bedtime as possible, or ask if you can change to a different medication.

Adjusting your nutritional, exercise, and sleep habits are all ways in which you can take an active part in reducing your pain and improving your health. It will improve your mental state too, because it feels good to take control of your life and see something good result from it.

Chapter 14

Alternative Healing Methods

There are many approaches to healing and wellness. Those of us who live in 21st-century America are most familiar with the *allopathic* approach used by medical doctors. It uses medicine and other procedures to try to alleviate health problems. We will refer to this as "conventional" medicine. In addition to allopathic or conventional medicine, there are many other approaches to achieving wellness and balance in the body. Chiropractic, homeopathic, naturopathic, and traditional Chinese medicine are some of the better-known alternative healing practices. We will refer to all of these as "alternative" methods.

There is a significant difference in approach between conventional and alternative methods. If you are unaware of this difference, it is easy to misunderstand what each group of practitioners is doing. Conventional medicine usually identifies symptoms and dysfunctions and seeks to treat them as a means of restoring health to the body. Alternative healing methods usually seeks to restore the natural balance of the body to enable it to heal itself, and thus to resolve dysfunctions.

Restoring wellness or balance rather than treating symptoms

Most alternative healing methods assess the condition of your body and then make an effort to help restore it to a state of wellness, rather than treating bothersome symptoms as they arise. This may be done by reestablishing balance within the body's systems, by providing the body with the nutrition it needs to restore itself and fight off disease, or by strengthening various parts of the body.   Different alternative disciplines target different issues, but generally they all seek to restore wellness as a means of dealing with disease and its dysfunction.

This explains part of the misunderstanding that often occurs when people who are accustomed to conventional medicine first encounter alternative healing practices. Alternative methods tend to be slower in producing obvious improvements, because they are depending on the body to bring about the improvement, rather than using chemicals. But when that improvement occurs, it is generally sustainable without medication and therefore it lacks the side effects of medications. The improvement is a result of the body moving toward healing, not just a suppression of symptoms.

Give alternative methods enough time to impact your body

If you are accustomed to conventional medicine it may seem that alternative practitioners are failing to deal aggressively enough with your symptoms.   You may feel like you are not getting sufficient relief from their treatments. Generally alternative therapies require several visits to the practitioner or several therapy or exercise treatments that you perform yourself at home.   It may seem that they "just want to keep you coming to get your money." Yet if you realize the goal–to restore wellness and balance to your body so that your body can heal itself– it makes more sense.   The body may retain the benefit of the treatment for only a few hours or days initially, but if, with repeated treatments, the body maintains that benefit for days, weeks, or months without medication, then the slow start is worth it in the end.   You have restored health to your body without the side effects that medications bring, or the expense of taking them.

Although at times it may work, it is not a good idea to use alternative methods primarily to relieve symptoms if you aren't really concerned about the overall wellness of your body. This is very commonly done with nutritional supplements. Supplements can and do improve various problems, but their long-term effectiveness ultimately still depends on having balance in the body.

The bonus of alternative practices is that their aim is to restore health to your body so you won't have symptoms. Providing your body with what it needs to heal itself is generally more effective in the long run than taking medication to cover up some symptoms.

Symptoms can be part of healing

The body has an amazing capacity to heal itself, especially if it is given what it needs to do so. Drugs frequently interrupt this process. It is true that they reduce symptoms, but the lessening of bothersome symptoms does not necessarily indicate healing. Often it is just a sign of the interruption in the body's natural way of dealing with a problem. For instance, reducing a fever by taking aspirin or Tylenol makes a patient more comfortable, but the fever is really one of the body's ways of fighting off a problem. It burns it up. If you are willing to put up with a fever (provided that it is not excessive), it may be more helpful to your body to rest and let the fever do its work than to take something to reduce the fever.

This may sound strange to you because you have become accustomed to taking medicine to reduce symptoms. This allows you to be more comfortable and to continue your normal routine even while your body is trying to fight off a problem. However this causes dual problems for your body.

Not only are its normal mechanisms for fighting disease being interfered with by the medication, but you are also staying active rather than resting to allow your body to utilize its energy for healing.

It is common to think that you can't let illness interrupt your schedule. Medication has allowed this mentality to develop. For instance, before Imodium was available, people didn't go anywhere if they were having trouble with diarrhea. Now it is often possible to pop a pill and go on with your day. But being able to stay active and being well are two very different things.

Which is your priority – your body or your schedule?

Until you grasp the difference in approaches it may be difficult to work successfully with alternative healing methods. But once you can distinguish for yourself the difference between allowing your body to heal and suppressing symptoms so you can stay active, you may benefit greatly from alternative approaches. It is appropriate to continue to use medication, but the point is that it is better to be an advocate for your *body*, and not just for your *schedule*. Ultimately a healthy body will allow you to do more anyway. But to have and maintain a healthy body, you will need to schedule time for it daily: time to relax, time to eat right, time to exercise, and time to allow it to deal with illness as it occurs.

Integrative Medicine Clinics

The conventional medical profession has increasingly been acknowledging the significance of alternative practices in treating chronic pain and other health issues. In fact, in recent years, *integrative medicine* clinics have been opening across the US. These clinics are run by MDs who are striving to combine the best ideas and practices of conventional and alternative approaches in order to maximize the body's potential for healing itself. The patient is evaluated and his history is taken. After the patient leaves, the physician meets with a group of practitioners and creates an individualized treatment plan for the patient, using appropriate therapies and treatments available at that clinic. At the next appointment, the physician reviews the plan with the patient. Then the patient begins to implement the plan by working with the appropriate practitioners or instructors. Therapies offered at each clinic vary, but they include some of the following:

Acupuncture
Biofeedback
Cranio-sacral therapy
Chiropractic
Energy medicine
Herbal medicine
Homeopathy
Hypnotherapy
Massage and bodywork
Mindfulness-based stress reduction
Mind-body medicine
Naturopathic medicine
Nutritional counseling
Osteopathic manipulation
Psychotherapy
Relaxation therapy

Traditional Chinese medicine
Yoga and other movement therapies

You may not have had the opportunity to use the services of an Integrative Medicine clinic, but you can learn some important ideas simply by knowing that they exist. You can see that there are many valid approaches to wellness and healing. You can also see that each health practitioner is trained in only one or, at the most, a few of the many treatment options available. So it is reasonable to assume that you may have to work with more than one practitioner, and there may be more than one therapy option that would be helpful for you. In fact, the body frequently responds best to a combination of treatments. At this point it is easy to short-circuit mentally. Who will supervise this "combination of treatments" Who will pay for them?? Take one thing at a time. Right now you are only trying to broaden your horizons and develop a slightly different way of approaching your quest for wellness.

Educate yourself

You can learn about some of the alternative therapies available by reading on the Internet, getting a book from the library, or talking with friends who have been successfully treated with alternative medicines. Then talk to your primary care physician before implementing alternative therapies. It is also very important to make sure that the alternative practitioner you are considering is certified and has successfully helped other patients with conditions similar to yours.

Interestingly enough, a recent survey found that more than a third of U.S. adults now use some form of alternative or complementary medicine. Chronic pain is the most frequent reason that people look beyond conventional medicine to alternative treatments for help. The National Center for

Complementary and Alternative Medicine is a division of the National Institutes of Health. Here are the five categories of complementary and alternative medicine it delineates:

- **Alternative medical systems** –such as acupuncture and traditional Chinese medicine.
- **Mind body interventions** –such as meditation and guided imagery.
- **Manipulating and adjusting the body** –this would include massage and chiropractic.
- **Biologically based therapies** –this would include herbs, vitamins and nutritional supplements used to promote healing.
- **Energy therapies** –this includes techniques that use energy fields to promote healing.

The acceptance of alternative treatments varies greatly within the conventional medical world. One doctor may be open to a certain treatment and may have found it to be helpful for his or her patients. The next doctor you work with may not be open at all to that same treatment. Much of the reason for this discrepancy is that there isn't a lot of scientific evidence to support the effectiveness of alternative treatments. In part, this is because there isn't funding to pay for the studies necessary to prove the effectiveness.

In the world of conventional medicine, many of the trial studies are funded by pharmaceutical companies who would profit greatly from the approval of the new drugs, so they are willing to spend the money to pay for the tests necessary to patent the drug. In the world of alternative medicine, many of the practices are hundreds or even thousands of years old. Testing their effectiveness won't result in patents or profit for any company.

Despite these challenges, alternative therapies are a good option for chronic pain. Conventional medicine recognizes chronic pain as one of the most difficult areas to treat. Taking pain medication for years or decades just doesn't work very well. The American Medical Association has acknowledged that chiropractic care is frequently more successful for low back pain than surgery is. Prayerfully consider alternative therapies. Educate yourself, talk to friends. *Your body will thank you!*

Chapter 15

My Personal Pain Journey

This book is the outpouring of my heart and mind from my more-than-15 years of living with severe chronic pain. It has shaped and changed my life. Although I never would have asked for such a journey, my life is better for it.

Somewhere in 1992 I started developing neck pain. This became a stiff neck and stiff and aching shoulders. Before long, I developed carpal tunnel in my right wrist. I struggled to continue using the computer to write Bible studies and arrange handbell music, two of my favorite pastimes. By 1994 it was becoming difficult for me to drive because my neck was so stiff I could hardly turn it to look for traffic.

In early 1995 I started working with a chiropractor. The net result was good, but it came at a price. It seems that every adjustment he made improved my mobility, but also aggravated my muscles. During that time my medical doctor commented to me once that I had myofascial pain. He never suggested a treatment plan for it or even told me what it was.

In April of 1996 my life changed dramatically. After a weekend trip in a 15-passenger van with the youth choir from our church, I developed sharp pains in my head. I had to lie down every two or three hours regardless of where I was, because the pain was so great that I couldn't stay upright.

My chiropractor worked on me for 2 or 3 weeks without any real progress, so he recommended that I see a neurologist. The neurologist ordered the first of numerous tests. Nothing definitive was found. By this time I had sharp shooting pains going down my arms. I was taking anti-inflammatory medication, using a home traction set, and following all the advice my doctors had given me, but by July I was losing strength in my arm muscles and my reflexes were diminishing. Finally, an MRI of my neck showed herniated discs at two levels (between two sets of vertebrae).

During this first phase of my pain journey I struggled to try to continue my normal life. I didn't want to "give in" to pain. I was determined to conquer it. I had no idea what chronic pain was. The first time someone used that term in relation to my situation, I actually went home and looked up the word "chronic" in a dictionary so I could figure out what chronic pain was.

Surgery

Conservative measures weren't helping. (This is another new term I learned. Conservative measures are non-invasive procedures or treatments other than surgery). The pain and associated problems were steadily increasing, so surgery seemed like the best option. In August of 1996 I had a discectomy and fusion surgery at two levels of my neck (plain English translation: discs were removed between two sets of vertebrae in my neck. Bone that had been taken from my hip bone was inserted between the vertebrae. The bones pieces were expected to all fuse together, and to prevent more nerves from being pinched.)

I vividly remember waking up in the recovery room with excruciating pain across the back of my skull, which was nowhere near the incision or where my pain had been prior to the surgery. The pain was so intense that as soon as I was moved to my room I asked for the bed to be raised so I could sit up. I simply could not stand to have a pillow touch my head. The hospital staff was hesitant to respond to my requests for more pain medication. My description of the pain seemed unlikely, I suppose. I was unable to sleep at night or rest comfortably during the day.

Things did not get any better once I got home. The bones fused perfectly and the incision healed without problems. But my pain seemed only to increase. The surgeon dismissed me because as far as he was concerned, I was okay. But he did refer me to a physical therapist.

The process of completing my initial P.T. examination aggravated my pain to the point that I was in tears. All this was so out of character for me. I have a very high pain threshold and I am not a complainer. I couldn't even recognize myself.

The exercises my physical therapist gave me to strengthen my neck muscles only seemed to create more problems instead of helping me. Fortunately, she was a very sensitive and skilled therapist and was determined to find a way to help me. Her encouragement became essential to my existence. (I continue to seek her wise counsel. She is one of the people I credit for the quality of my wellness today.)

By three months after my surgery I was desperate for help. I went back to my primary care physician to see what he could offer me. His opinion was that I had postoperative depression, and he recommended anti-depressants. I had stopped taking the pain medication the surgeons had given me because it had minimal effect on the pain and just seemed to make me feel groggy and decrease my ability to cope with the pain. I was not eager to take more medication. I also knew that the pain I was experiencing might depress me, but it certainly was not the result of depression. On my own initiative I was getting acupuncture treatments, which seemed to help more than the medications.

I was not experienced in visiting doctors and working with doctors' offices. Nor did I know how to use pain medication to deal with chronic pain, as I had never experienced it before. My approach was to wait until I couldn't stand the pain before taking any medication, which only made things worse.

My physical therapist and chiropractor were key in guiding me through this time and helping me to begin to learn how to deal with both chronic pain and the medical world. Because physical therapists, acupuncturists, massage therapists, and chiropractors spend time working with your body, there is time to talk to them as they work. They often seek out additional information about your activity levels, mood, etc. This exchange of information can be invaluable for both you and them. New angles about the cause of your pain or ways to treat it may surface. They also have time to give you additional hints on how to live with your pain.

I began to learn that I was responsible for my health, not my doctor. I took the initiative to find another primary care physician. She was a better fit for me, as she specialized in pain and had fibromyalgia herself. She identified a massive problem with myofascial pain and the triggers associated with it. (Myofascial pain results from tender points–trigger points–that develop in muscles due to a variety of reasons.) We tried rounds of injections followed by physical therapy to try to get rid of the triggers. This helped, but the triggers came back very quickly. This indicated to my doctor that there was another problem that was perpetuating the myofascial pain. We tested for multiple sclerosis, myasthenia gravis, and many other syndromes and diseases. I had test after test and was referred to doctor after doctor. My pain continued to get worse and we were unable to identify the root problem.

The diagnosis

Finally, after two years of testing and thousands of dollars spent for tests, doctors' appointments, medications, and therapies, one procedure–a stellate ganglion block–had a positive result. It showed that I had reflex sympathetic dystrophy (RSD). (This is also called complex regional pain syndrome. It is a malfunction of the sympathetic nervous system, usually caused by an injury or some other type of trauma.) I was relieved to finally have a diagnosis. However I was told that that RSD is very treatable in its early stages. And as long as it is treated within the first six months it is generally reversible. By this time, however, I had been suffering with it for two years.

We started to treat the RSD aggressively but the results were not encouraging. The anesthesiologist who first diagnosed the RSD felt that he was not getting the response he had hoped for from the blocks. So he referred me to a pain specialist. The pain specialist tried a somewhat more aggressive approach, putting a catheter in my back so that we could more easily do repeated blocks. But before long, the scarring from the catheters caused so much pain that we could no longer continue the treatments.

In the three-and-a-half years that I worked with that pain specialist, we tried over fifty medications to see what would help me. I am very grateful to this man. He was the one who finally put together the protocol that began to turn the course of my pain. But the process was grueling. Each new medication jerked my body in a different direction. Often the side effects caused more problem than the benefits I received from the medication. Ultimately we found three or four medications that did help. (I still take three of these.)

By this time my pain had escalated to where I had virtually no life. I had stopped all activities. Frequently I was in too much pain to drive or even to fix food for my family. I left the house for doctors' appointments and occasionally church when I felt well enough. I was also seriously depressed.

I continued to find meaning in life through my faith in God. The one activity I seemed to be able to do was to talk (usually on the phone) with other people who were struggling with pain, and to share with them some practical tips I was learning, as well as the insights I was gaining from God's Word on how He uses pain to shape us, perfect us, and cause us to lean on Him.

I was having difficulty wearing clothing. I could only wear loose-fitting pajama-like outfits, because anything else hurt me. I couldn't stand to have air blowing on me and it was very difficult for me to adjust to cold or hot conditions. The RSD had created hypersensitivity in me towards many things. I was also very sensitive to visual and auditory stimulation. I needed to spend a lot of time in a quiet room with my eyes closed.

Spinal Cord Stimulator implant

My pain specialist recommended trying a spinal cord stimulator. I was quite convinced that I had already tried every kind of stimulator in existence, but this particular stimulator was implanted, rather than worn externally. The trial seemed promising, so I had the surgery to implant it. The surgery set me back quite a bit, as it aggravated my myofascial pain. But the sensitivity to touch that I had developed due to my RSD diminished significantly after the stimulator was implanted.

My body was also very rundown by this point. I was developing problems in other areas of my body just from the strain of all the pain. By the summer of 2000 I finally had to start taking narcotic pain medication because I could not bear the pain any longer. We planned another surgery to implant the stimulator electrode higher up my spinal cord to help the neck pain. Ultimately this lowered my pain to livable levels, but the surgery was very invasive and it again aggravated the myofascial pain terribly.

A full year after that surgery, I was still recovering from it. Finally we tried massive botox injections in the muscles that had been aggravated by the surgery. This was helpful, but initially the change in muscle tension caused many of the muscles we hadn't injected to spasm. This caused new excruciating pain. After a few months things had calmed down and I truly began to improve. However by this time my body was quite depleted in many ways and my muscles simply would not strengthen.

For a couple of years I took a pillow and blanket with me to every doctor appointment. Because I wasn't able to sit in a chair while I waited for my appointment, I had to lie down somewhere. If there wasn't an extra room I could use, I wrapped myself up in a corner of the waiting room. I couldn't stay upright very long and I couldn't tolerate the air conditioning. There were months when I could barely eat because I was in so much pain that I felt sick to my stomach all the time.

Help from alternative medicine

I sought the help of a naturopathic doctor. She did some tests and discovered that my amino acid levels were extremely low, which would explain why my muscles wouldn't strengthen. I began supplements and started to see a small but immediate improvement. What an incredible blessing! The improvement continued slowly but steadily.

I was also extremely depressed by this time. Several of my medical doctors said they simply couldn't help me anymore. My naturopathic doctor was quite sure she could help, but she said that it could take six months before there would be significant improvement. In fact it took more than six months before the depression was under control, but within one month I could already see some improvement.

Another therapy that helped me immeasurably was a simple one: soaking in a hot tub. I stumbled on warm water therapy at the very lowest point in my pain journey when nothing seemed to help. One hot August day, at the urging of a visiting relative (who is an MD) I got into a friend's swimming pool. I immediately felt relief from my neck and head pain. The buoyancy of the water took pressure off my neck, and the warmth (the pool was 90 plus degrees) soothed my muscles. I returned to the pool as often as I could. Soon my parents offered to buy us a hot tub. I have soaked in it almost daily ever since.

Finding life once again

Finally in the fall of 2002 I began to reenter life. I committed myself to attending a weekly class at church for the first time in four years. I tried to make it to church every Sunday for the first time in many years. This meant that on the days I was going to be out, I had to plan my entire day, and sometimes the day before, around being rested for my outing. It was a still monumental struggle just to leave the house to go to class once a week. To help support my neck I had a special chair at church to sit in. I would wrap a scarf around my neck if the room was too cold. Frequently I would need to stand in the back of the room so I could walk around every now and then, because I couldn't sit in one position for two hours.

Slowly, as I began to feel better, I was determined to get off the narcotics. In 2001 I began weaning myself off of them by very gradually lowering the dose every time my pain seemed to allow it. Finally, in the fall of 2003, I was able to stop taking the narcotic and to substitute a moderate amount of another pain medication for it. That was a milestone for me. The narcotics had caused me to be groggy. Often I began a sentence and found myself talking about something completely different by the end of the sentence. I simply did not want to live that kind of life.

The protocol that I had worked out with the help of the 6 to 8 medical professionals that I regularly saw included:

- *my routine prescriptions*
- *creams and patches for break-through pain*
- *numerous nutritional supplements taken daily*
- *cranio-sacral therapy every third week*
- *acupuncture every other week*
- *Chinese herbs as needed*
- *chiropractic care every other week*
- *daily walks*
- *daily exercises prescribed by my physical therapist*
- *daily time in the hot tub*
- *frequent use of hot packs during the day*
- *a short nap once or twice a day*
- *avoiding car travel as much as possible*
- *avoiding over stimulation (noisy environments, bright or moving lights, etc.)*

If I missed any one of these elements, my pain level would increase. We frequently tried reducing the dosage or eliminating a supplement or medication. Sometimes I was okay with the change, and sometimes it was clear that the treatment was helping me and shouldn't be changed. Through this experimenting with treatments and doses, I saw that each thing helped me and was worth the time and money spent on it. I had very knowledgeable and well-trained medical professionals guiding this process. The combination of all these elements lowered my pain enough that I was now able to do one, and occasionally two, activities outside the home on several days of the week.

Almost a decade later

Each year since 2003 (now it is 2010) I have been able to do a little bit more with a little bit less struggle. I still push my limit and find I that have upset the delicate balance between activity and rest. My pain causes me to appreciate everything that I am able to do, and also to evaluate every possible activity to determine if it is worth the toll it will take on my body.

I still take three prescription medications routinely and follow most of the rest of the same protocol. Occasionally I miss a dose of my pain medication and within a few hours, my pain is so intense that I can barely force myself to get up out of a chair. It is a good reminder of my need for the medications as well as for the rest of my treatment plan. I have discovered that when my pain levels begin to increase, I need to adjust my lifestyle, not increase my medications.

Lifestyle changes have been the key to my recovery. This book is what I live by. I wrote it because I found myself repeating its principles, over and over again, to various people God has put in my path. This is the prescription that God gave me. Every thought presented in this book, God worked out with me in my own life as I struggled to make sense out of my pain.

God has changed every aspect of my life. I simply don't do a lot of things I used to do. I would love to do them, but the price is just too high to make it worth it. But I have found lots of other satisfying things to do with my life. I believe that God has used my pain to direct my life. It is my desire to work with Him and not against Him.

Today, I am very active at church, teaching two women's Bible studies every week and assisting my husband with two more classes. I enjoy spending time with our five-year-old grandson. I do quite a bit of sewing, gardening, and writing, as well as mentoring and teaching. I try to keep one or two days each week very quiet, as this "down time" is important for maintaining balance in my body. I only see my cranio-sacral therapist and chiropractor once a month now. Instead of living a little bit of life between medical treatments and appointments, I now live a life and fit my daily exercise routine and occasional medical appointments into it. I am very grateful to God for the good life I enjoy. I hope to continue to improve and to be able to do some things that I presently can't do.

In conclusion

I hope that my pain journey helps to validate your pain journey. Each one is very real, but very hard to measure. Therefore we are left to wonder if anyone understands or cares. I could not possibly have survived these years without the continuous, loving care of my husband. Many friends and medical professionals also spent hours encouraging and listening to me. For several years, one very precious friend of mine spent one day a week driving me to physical therapy, helping me run errands and fixing me lunch in the middle of the day while I rested. She was a blessing beyond description.

I pray that God will provide people in your life to listen, help, care, and try to understand. God has truly provided for me in the midst of this journey. I know that it is His desire to provide for you too. I pray that you will find Him faithful *in the midst* of your pain journey.